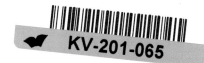
Megan Whitnall
Des R. Richardson

Iron Metabolism, Chelation and Disease

Megan Whitnall
Des R. Richardson

Iron Metabolism, Chelation and Disease

Iron and Iron Chelation in Disease

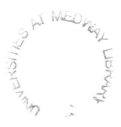

LAP LAMBERT Academic Publishing

Impressum / Imprint
Bibliografische Information der Deutschen Nationalbibliothek: Die Deutsche Nationalbibliothek verzeichnet diese Publikation in der Deutschen Nationalbibliografie; detaillierte bibliografische Daten sind im Internet über http://dnb.d-nb.de abrufbar.
Alle in diesem Buch genannten Marken und Produktnamen unterliegen warenzeichen-, marken- oder patentrechtlichem Schutz bzw. sind Warenzeichen oder eingetragene Warenzeichen der jeweiligen Inhaber. Die Wiedergabe von Marken, Produktnamen, Gebrauchsnamen, Handelsnamen, Warenbezeichnungen u.s.w. in diesem Werk berechtigt auch ohne besondere Kennzeichnung nicht zu der Annahme, dass solche Namen im Sinne der Warenzeichen- und Markenschutzgesetzgebung als frei zu betrachten wären und daher von jedermann benutzt werden dürften.

Bibliographic information published by the Deutsche Nationalbibliothek: The Deutsche Nationalbibliothek lists this publication in the Deutsche Nationalbibliografie; detailed bibliographic data are available in the Internet at http://dnb.d-nb.de.
Any brand names and product names mentioned in this book are subject to trademark, brand or patent protection and are trademarks or registered trademarks of their respective holders. The use of brand names, product names, common names, trade names, product descriptions etc. even without a particular marking in this works is in no way to be construed to mean that such names may be regarded as unrestricted in respect of trademark and brand protection legislation and could thus be used by anyone.

Coverbild / Cover image: www.ingimage.com

Verlag / Publisher:
LAP LAMBERT Academic Publishing
ist ein Imprint der / is a trademark of
AV Akademikerverlag GmbH & Co. KG
Heinrich-Böcking-Str. 6-8, 66121 Saarbrücken, Deutschland / Germany
Email: info@lap-publishing.com

Herstellung: siehe letzte Seite /
Printed at: see last page
ISBN: 978-3-8454-7760-2

Zugl. / Approved by: Sydney, University of Sydney, Diss., 2011

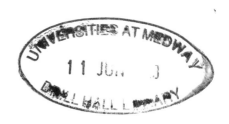

TABLE OF CONTENTS

CHAPTER 1

GENERAL INTRODUCTION 7

1.1 THE BIOLOGY AND IMPORTANCE OF IRON 8

1.2 PHYSIOLOGICAL IRON METABOLISM 10

1.2.1 The Source of Iron..10

1.2.2 Dietary Iron Absorption 10

1.2.3 Intracellular Iron Metabolism..11

1.2.3.1 Serum Iron Transport and Cellular Iron Uptake 11

1.2.3.2 Cytosolic Iron Trafficking and the Intracellular Labile Iron 13

1.2.3.3 Cytosolic Iron Storage...14

1.2.4.1 Mitochondrial Iron Uptake..18

1.2.4.2 Mitochondrial Iron Storage...19

1.2.4.3 Iron Sulfur Cluster Synthesis 20

1.2.4.4 Haem Synthesis..22

1.3 IRON HOMEOSTASIS 24

1.3.1 Cellular Iron Homeostasis 24

1.3.2 Systemic Iron Homeostasis 27

1.4 IRON IN DISEASE 28

1.4.1 Alzheimer's Disease..30

1.4.2 Parkinson's Disease..31

1.4.3 Friedreich's Ataxia 32

1.5 IRON CHELATORS FOR THE TREATMENT DISEASE...........................35

1.5.1 Iron Chelation for the Treatment of Cancer 36

1.5.2 Properties to be Considered in the Design of Clinically Useful Iron Chelators...37

1.5.3 Desferrioxamine 40

1.5.4 Pyridoxal isonicotinoyl hydrazone 41

1.6 SPECIFIC OBJECTIVES 42

CHAPTER 2

MATERIALS AND METHODS 44

2.1 REAGENTS 45

2.1.1 Chemicals 45

2.1.2 Buffers and Solutions 45

2.1.3 Diferric-Transferrin 46

2.2 ANIMALS **46**

2.2.1 Monitoring and Ethics 46

2.2.2 Necroscopy 47

2.3 ANALYSIS OF BIOLOGICAL ANIMAL PARAMETERS **47**

2.3.1 Haematological Indices 47

2.3.2 Tissue Iron Estimation...47

2.3.3 Histology 48

2.4 DETECTION OF mRNA USING RT-PCR.....................................**49**

2.4.1 Isolation of RNA from Animal Tissues...49

2.4.2 Reverse Transcriptase-Polymerase Chain Reaction 49

2.5 DETECTION OF PROTEIN USING WESTERN BLOT ANALYSIS **50**

2.5.1 Extraction of Protein from Animal Tissues...................................50

2.5.2 Western Blot Analysis 51

2.6 IRP-RNA BINDING ACTIVITY..**52**

2.6.1 Extraction of Protein from Animal Tissue 52

2.6.2 Gel Retardation Analysis...52

2.7 IN VIVO ADMINISTRATION OF ^{59}FE AND CELLULAR

FRACTIONATION..**53**

2.8 ANALYSIS OF RESULTS AND DATA **53**

2.8.1 Densitometry 53

2.8.2 Statistics..53

CHAPTER 3

A CLASS OF IRON CHELATORS WITH A WIDE SPECTRUM OF

POTENT ANTI-TUMOUR ACTIVITY THAT OVERCOME

RESISTANCE TO CHEMOTHERAPEUTICS **55**

3.1 INTRODUCTION **56**

3.2 MATERIALS AND METHODS..**59**

3.2.1 Chelators and Cytotoxics..59

3.2.2 Cell culture 59

3.2.3 MTT Cell Proliferation Assay 60

2

3.2.4 Colony Formation Assay 61

3.2.5 Tumour Xenografts in Nude Mice and Chelator Administration 62

3.2.6 Serum Biochemistry and Blood Cell Morphology 63

3.2.7 Gene Expression Analysis 63

3.3 RESULTS **65**

3.3.1 DpT and PKIH Iron Chelators Show High Anti-proliferative Activity Against a Range of Tumour Cell Lines 65

3.3.2 Clonogenic Assays with Dp44mT 69

3.3.3 Dp44mT Retains Anti-proliferative Activity in Drug-Resistant Cell Lines ...69

3.3.4 Sensitivity of Tumour Cells to DpT Chelators is Independent of p53 Status 72

3.3.5 Dp44mT Markedly Inhibits the Growth of Human Tumour Xenografts *In Vivo* 72

3.3.5.1 Short-Term Studies 72

3.3.5.2 Long-Term Studies 73

3.3.6 Biological Assessment Following Chelator Treatment 75

3.3.7 Organ Weights and Tissue Iron Levels After Chelator Treatment 78

3.3.8 Effects of Chelators on Tissue Histology and Blood Cell Morphology 81

3.3.9 Effect of Iron Chelation on the Expression of Iron-Responsive Genes in the Tumour and Liver 84

3.4 DISCUSSION **87**

3.4.1 *In Vitro* Evaluation 87

3.4.2 *In Vivo* Evaluation 89

CHAPTER 4

CONDITIONAL FRATAXIN KNOCKOUT IN THE FRIEDREICH'S ATAXIA HEART: TREATMENT BY IRON CHELATION THERAPY AND ELUCIDATION OF MITOCHONDRIAL IRON LOADING PATHWAYS

LOADING PATHWAYS 93

4.1 INTRODUCTION **94**

4.2 MATERIALS AND METHODS **96**

4.2.1 Animals 96

4.2.2 Genotyping 96

4.2.3 Chelator Studies 97

4.2.4 RT-PCR Analysis 98

4.2.5 Western Analysis...99

4.2.6 Uptake and Intracellular Distribution of ^{59}Fe *In Vivo* 99

4.2.7 Native PAGE ^{59}Fe Autoradiography and Anion-Exchange

Chromatography 100

4.3 RESULTS..101

4.3.1 Altered Cardiac Iron Metabolism in the Mutant 101

4.3.2 IRP2-RNA Binding Activity is Increased in Mutant Heart.............105

4.3.3 Marked Alterations in Cytosolic ^{59}Fc Distribution within Ferritin in Mutant

Heart 109

4.3.4 Iron Chelation 112

4.3.4.1 Chelation Reduces Heart Iron in the Mutant 112

4.3.4.2 Growth After Chelation 115

4.3.4.3 Chelation Limits Heart Hypertrophy....................................115

4.4 DISCUSSION...118

CHAPTER 5

CONDITIONAL FRATAXIN KNOCKOUT IN THE FRIEDREICH'S

ATAXIA HEART: TREATMENT BY IRON SUPPLEMENTATION

AND DEMONSTRATION OF THE CARDIAC CONTROL OF

SYSTEMIC IRON METABOLISM 123

5.1 INTRODUCTION 124

5.2 MATERIALS AND METHODS..127

5.2.1 Animals and Genotyping...127

5.2.2 Dietary Iron Supplementation Studies..127

5.2.3 Western Analysis...127

5.2.4 Size-Exclusion Chromatography 128

5.2.5 Transmission Electron Microscopy...128

5.2.6 Magnetic Susceptibility Measurements..129

5.3 RESULTS..130

5.3.1 Iron Supplementation Delays Weight Loss and Limits Cardiac

Hypertrophy...130

5.3.1.1 Animal Growth After Iron Supplementation............................131

5.3.1.2 Cardiac Hypertrophy After Iron Supplementation 131

5.3.1.3 Organ Iron Content After Iron Supplementation 132

5.3.2 Effect of Iron Supplementation on Expression of Proteins in the Heart and Liver 134

5.3.2.1 Frataxin Deficiency Does Not Lead to the Normal Physiologic Response to Dietary Iron Loading in the Mutant Heart 134

5.3.2.2 RNA-Binding Activity of IRP2 is not Decreased in Mutants Hearts by Iron Loading 138

5.3.2.3 Systemic Effects in the Liver Following Frataxin Deletion in the Heart and Skeletal Muscle 141

5.3.3 Iron Accumulates in the Mutant Heart in a Unique Form 144

5.3.3.1 Marked Alterations Exist in ^{59}Fe Distribution in the Mutant Heart 145

5.3.3.2 Transmission Electron Microscopy Demonstrates Ferritin Iron Accumulation in the Mutant Liver and Non Ferritin Iron Accumulation in the Mutant Heart 149

5.3.3.3 Magnetic Susceptibility Measurements Demonstrate Anti-ferromagnetic Iron in the Mutant Heart is Not Present in Ferritin 150

5.4 DISCUSSION 154

5.4.1 Cytosolic Iron Deficiency and the Effect of Iron Supplementation Using a High Iron Diet 154

5.4.2 Conditional Frataxin Deletion in the Heart Leads to Systemic Alterations in Iron Metabolism 156

5.4.3 Iron Accumulation in the Mitochondrion of the Mutant Heart Does Not Occur as Ferritin 158

CHAPTER 6
GENERAL DISCUSSION AND FUTURE DIRECTIONS 161

6.1 DISCUSSION PRELUDE 162

6.2 A CLASS OF IRON CHELATORS WITH A WIDE SPECTRUM OF POTENT ANTI-TUMOUR ACTIVITY THAT OVERCOME RESISTANCE TO CHEMOTHERAPEUTICS 163

6.2.1 Significance and Summary of Principal Findings - Chapter 3 163

6.2.2 Subsequent Studies and Future Experiments Examining the Development of Iron Chelators as Cancer Therapeutics 165

6.2.2.1 The Anti-Metastatic Effect of Dp44mT 165

6.2.2.2 New Mechanisms of Action Justify Further Development of Dp44mT . 167

6.2.2.3 Pharmacokinetic Studies 168

6.2.2.4 Structure-Activity Analysis of Dp44mT 169

6.3 CONDITIONAL FRATAXIN KNOCKOUT IN THE FRIEDREICH'S ATAXIA HEART: TREATMENT BY IRON CHELATION THERAPY AND ELUCIDATION OF MITOCHONDRIAL IRON LOADING PATHWAYS ... 172

6.3.1 Significance and Summary of Principal Findings - Chapter 4 172

6.3.2 Future Studies Examining Intracellular Iron Trafficking Pathways in the MCK Mouse 175

6.3.2.1 Cellular Iron Uptake 175

6.3.2.2 Cytosolic Iron Transporters 176

6.3.2.3 Mitochondrial Iron Import 178

6.3.3 Future Studies Examining Chelation Therapy in the MCK Mouse.............179

6.3.3.1 Proof of Principle - Ensuring PIH Does Not Deplete the Cytosolic Compartment 179

6.3.3.2 Analogues of 2-Pyridylcarboxaldehyde Isonicotinoyl Hydrazone (PCIH) as Ligands for the Treatment of Friedreich's Ataxia 180

6.3.4 Future Studies Examining Neurodegeneration in Friedreich's Ataxia.........182

6.3.4.1 The Neuron-Specific Enolase Transgenic Mouse Model 182

6.3.4.2 Other Mouse Models of Friedreich's Ataxia 185

6.4 CONDITIONAL FRATAXIN KNOCKOUT IN THE FRIEDREICH'S ATAXIA HEART: TREATMENT BY IRON SUPPLEMENTATION AND DEMONSTRATION OF THE CARDIAC CONTROL OF SYSTEMIC IRON METABOLISM 187

6.4.1 Significance and Summary of Principal Findings – Chapter 5 187

6.4.2 Future Studies Examining Iron Supplementation Therapy 189

6.4.2.1 Iron Supplementation Using SIH-Fe 189

6.4.3 Identifying the Cause of Systemic Iron Overload in the MCK Mouse 190

6.4.3.1 Hepcidin and Ferroportin1 191

6.4.3.2 Protein Regulators of Hepcidin Expression 193

6.4.4 Identifying the Form of Iron in the Mitochondrion of the MCK Mouse......195

6.5 CONCLUDING REMARKS...196

CHAPTER 7

REFERENCES 197

CHAPTER 1

GENERAL INTRODUCTION

THIS CHAPTER IS ADAPTED FROM:

Whitnall M and Richardson DR (2006) Iron: A new target for pharmacological intervention in neurodegenerative diseases. *Semin Paediatric Neurol* 13(3):186-97. *Invited review.*

Richardson DR, Huang ML, **Whitnall M**, Becker EM, Ponka P, Rahmanto YS. The ins and outs of mitochondrial iron-loading: the metabolic defect in Friedreich's ataxia. *J Mol Med* (2010) 88(4):323-9. *Invited review.*

Richardson DR, Lane DJ, Becker EM, Huang ML, **Whitnall M**, Rahmanto YS, Sheftel AD, Ponka P. Mitochondrial iron trafficking and the integration of iron metabolism between mitochondrion and cytosol. *Proc Natl Acad Sci USA* (2010) 107(24):10775-82. *Invited review.*

1.1 THE BIOLOGY AND IMPORTANCE OF IRON

Iron is an integral and essential part of daily life and arguably, one of the most important transition metals of the body. This is highlighted by the need for iron and iron-containing molecules to facilitate key metabolic reactions (Rouault and Tong, 2008, Sheftel and Lill, 2009). For example, iron is required by the iron-containing enzyme, ribonucleotide reductase, during the rate-limiting step of DNA synthesis (Thelander and Reichard, 1979). Furthermore, an absence of iron in cell cycle progression, arrests cells at the G1/S interface and induces apoptosis (Brodie et al., 1993, Richardson and Milnes, 1997).

Within the energy producing environment of the mitochondrion, iron is required for iron-sulfur cluster (ISC) (Muhlenhoff and Lill, 2000) and haem synthesis (Ponka, 1997). In turn, ISC and haem prosthetic groups are essential components of many metallo-proteins. Notable examples of proteins requiring ISCs include: (i) respiratory chain complexes I and II, also known as NADH dehydrogenase and succinate dehydrogenase, respectively (Rouault and Tong, 2008); (ii) mitochondrial aconitase of the tricarboxylic acid cycle (Rouault and Tong, 2008); and (iii) isopropylmalate isomerase, which is required for amino acid synthesis (Sheftel and Lill, 2009). Notable haem-requiring proteins include: (i) haemoglobin, which is involved in oxygen transport (Sheftel and Lill, 2009); (ii) myoglobin, which is involved in oxygen storage (Sheftel and Lill, 2009); and (iii) c-type cytochromes, which are involved in respiration (Kuchar and Hausinger, 2004). Superfluous to these ubiquitous pathways, the unique environment of the brain harbors additional iron requirements to necessitate the synthesis of myelin and neurotransmitters (Burdo and Connor, 2003).

8

Indeed, many of these diverse processes are a derivative of iron's unique ability to redox cycle *via* electron exchange. Iron has two stable oxidation states, *i.e.,* ferrous iron or iron(II), and ferric iron or iron(III) (Kalinowski and Richardson, 2005). The ability of iron to shuttle between these two forms, acting as an electron acceptor or donor, catalyses biochemical reactions such as those mentioned above (Kalinowski and Richardson, 2005). Paradoxically though, this redox property also renders iron a highly toxic metal. Interactions between iron and oxygen metabolites, or 'Fenton chemistry', generates reactive oxygen species (ROS), which readily react with some of the cells most important biomolecules, including proteins, lipids and DNA (Halliwell and Gutteridge, 2007, Halliwell and Gutteridge, 1999). Ensuing cellular damage and 'oxidative stress' involves lipid peroxidation, protein aggregation and unfolding, and DNA and mitochondrial oxidation, which can impair cellular functions and ultimately lead to cell death (Barnham et al., 2004, Polla, 1999).

The toxicity of iron, when present in excess of physiological requirements, is evident in numerous pathological conditions. Iron accumulation and ensuing oxidative stress have been associated with the common inherited disease, β-Thalassemia (Olivieri and Brittenham, 1997) and the severe cardio- and neuro-degenerative disease, Friedreich's ataxia (Calabrese et al., 2005, Schulz et al., 2000). Conversely, iron deficiency can also be detrimental to the cell, due to the countless cellular processes which are dependent on iron to function. To prevent the consequences of iron overload or deficiency, the body possesses an extensive collection of proteins and pathways by which it can regulate iron homeostasis. These important iron metabolism processes, and how we have come to understand them through the study of disease, are integrally discussed below.

1.2 PHYSIOLOGICAL IRON METABOLISM

1.2.1 The Source of Iron

For the healthy individual, total body iron approximates 50 mg/kg (Munoz et al., 2009). The lack of an effective mechanism for excreting iron (McCance and Widdowson, 1938) means that iron levels must be impeccably managed *via* regulation of dietary iron uptake and conservation of tissue iron stores. The large proportion of iron for cellular use, is sourced from internal iron storage sinks such as the cellular iron storage protein, ferritin, and is recycled by macrophages which phagocytose senescent erythrocytes to release iron from haem (Dunn et al., 2007). Additionally, a small portion (0.5-2 mg/day) is also obtained externally from dietary iron absorption through the enterocytes of the duodenum, primarily to replace iron lost from daily blood losses and epithelial cell shedding (Sharp and Srai, 2007, Munoz et al., 2009).

1.2.2 Dietary Iron Absorption

The process of dietary iron absorption involves the uptake of iron from the lumen of the gut, transit across the apical membrane, transcellular trafficking, and release through the basolateral membrane of the enterocyte, after which iron is incorporated into the serum for cellular distribution (Munoz et al., 2009).

The uptake of iron across the apical enterocyte membrane occurs *via* two different pathways. Dietary non-haem iron is not in a readily bioavailable form, and must be reduced before it can cross the apical enterocyte membrane. While this role can be performed by the ferrireductase,

10

duodenal cytochrome-b *in vitro* (McKie, 2008, McKie et al., 2001), accurate studies using *duodenal cytochrome-b* knockout models are required before we can rule out the presence of other ferrireductases (Frazer et al., 2005, Gunshin et al., 2005). After this reduction process, iron is transported into the cytoplasm by the divalent metal transporter 1 (DMT1) (Mims and Prchal, 2005).

On the other hand, dietary iron found in haem, is absorbed *via* receptor-mediated endocytosis after haem binds to the apical membrane-bound protein, haem carrier protein-1 (Shayeghi et al., 2005). Once internalised into the enterocyte, iron is liberated from haem by haem oxygenase 1 (Hmox1) (Dunn et al., 2007).

Within the cytoplasm of the enterocyte, iron which has been imported by DMT1 or liberated from haem, is metabolised *via* a common intracellular pathway as discussed in Section 1.2.3 below. At the basolateral membrane, iron is transported out of the enterocyte by ferroportin1 (Donovan et al., 2005). Ferroportin1 is expressed in all iron-exporting cells and is the only known mechanism of cellular iron efflux (Troadec et al., 2010). Deletion of ferroportin1 is embryonically lethal, and conditional knockout of *ferroportin1* leads to increased iron storage in enterocytes, macrophages and hepatocytes (Donovan et al., 2005). Thus it plays a critical role in iron homeostasis, regulating intracellular cytosolic iron levels and export of iron to the serum (Troadec et al., 2010).

1.2.3 Intracellular Iron Metabolism

1.2.3.1 Serum Iron Transport and Cellular Iron Uptake

Under normal physiological circumstances, the movement of iron throughout the serum is tightly regulated. After it exits the enterocyte, iron binds to the serum glycoprotein, transferrin (Tf) (Morgan 1981). Each Tf molecule is capable of binding two atoms of iron, with exceptionally high affinity (Aisen et al., 1978, Morgan, 1981), producing a diferric-Tf complex. High affinity iron binding, and the abundance of Tf in the serum, means that little, if any, iron enters the circulation as unbound and potentially toxic 'free' iron (Anderson and Vulpe, 2009). At the plasma cell membrane, circulating diferric-Tf binds to the cell surface protein, transferrin receptor 1 (TfR1) (Richardson and Ponka, 1997). Binding induces receptor-mediated endocytosis, which internalises the Tf-TfR1 iron complex (Richardson and Ponka, 1997), as demonstrated in Figure 1.1. Following a reduction in endosomal pH, iron is released from the complex and transported into the cytoplasm *via* DMT1, while iron-free, apo-Tf-TfR1, is recycled back to the cell surface and Tf returned to the circulation (Gunshin et al., 1997, Morgan, 1981, Ponka et al., 1998).

While high affinity TfR1-mediated iron uptake represents the primary and most efficient means by which cells take up iron (Richardson and Ponka, 1997), a number of other iron uptake pathways have been identified. Hepatocytes in particular express high levels of the TfR1 homologue, transferrin receptor 2 (TfR2) (Kawabata et al., 2001, Kawabata et al., 1999). Like TfR1, TfR2 also internalises Tf-bound iron by a receptor-mediated endocytic process (Graham et al., 2008), although the affinity of this pathway is up to 30-fold lower than that of TfR1 (West et al., 2000). Interestingly, deletion of TfR2 does not have a substantial impact on Tf-bound iron uptake in the liver of *TfR2$^{-/-}$* mice, and indeed, the primary role of TfR2 is currently thought to be in systemic iron regulation as opposed to cellular iron uptake (Chua et al., 2010).

Additionally, the presence of non-transferrin-bound iron (NTBI) has been detected in the sera of patients with iron overload diseases such as thalassemia (Esposito et al., 2003, Hershko et al., 1978) and haemochromatosis (Gosriwatana et al., 1999, Loreal et al., 2000). The pathological appearance of circulating NTBI has been associated with major ingression of iron into cells by unregulated routes (Cabantchik et al., 2005). The instance of NTBI is generally thought to occur when iron entering the serum exceeds the iron-binding capacity of Tf (Anderson and Vulpe, 2009). This may be due to unregulated dietary iron absorption, or defects in iron-handling proteins (Anderson and Vulpe, 2009). For example, a congenital deficiency in Tf in the rare iron overload condition, atransferrinemia, underlies the appearance of NTBI and causes hemosiderosis in organs such as the liver, heart and endocrine organs (Anderson and Vulpe, 2009, Beutler et al., 2000).

1.2.3.2 Cytosolic Iron Trafficking and the Intracellular Labile Iron

After it is released from the classical Tf-TfR1 endosome (Figure 1.1), the pathways that traffic cytosolic iron to intracellular organelles and compartments, are not fully understood. Initially, iron is thought to enter a poorly characterised cytosolic compartment known as the intracellular labile iron pool (LIP) (Richardson and Ponka, 1997). The molecular nature and composition of the LIP has not been comprehensively elucidated. Low (Jacobs, 1977) and high (Petrak and Vyoral, 2001) molecular weight ligands, which bear chelatable forms of iron (Konijn et al., 1999), have been suggested to be present. Presuming its existence, the LIP most likely functions to transiently bind iron after cellular iron uptake, before incorporation into other intracellular compartments (Greenberg and

Wintrobe, 1946, Konijn et al., 1999) such as ferritin and the mitochondrion (Figure 1.1).

Recent studies are challenging the idea of the LIP. Fluorescent confocal and transmission electron microscopy have demonstrated that in the developing erythroid cell, there is a direct interorganeller transfer of iron from Tf-containing endosomes to the mitochondrion (Sheftel et al., 2007). During transient physical contact between the endosome and mitochondrion, iron is delivered directly from compartment to compartment, by-passing the LIP, in a mechanism colloquially referred to as the 'kiss and run' hypothesis (Sheftel et al., 2007). The molecular framework of proteins and docking complexes reasoned to facilitate this compartmental iron transfer were not identified at the time, but studies using the haemoglobin-deficit (*hbd*) mouse, identified the Sec15l1 exocyst protein as a possible candidate (Sheftel et al., 2007). Characteristically, erythrocytes of *hbd* mice, exhibit decreased haemoglobin synthesis and recycling of endosomal-Tf, due to a mutation in *Sec15l1*, which is a homologue of the yeast gene that encodes the vesicle docking protein, SEC15 (Lim et al., 2005, White et al., 2005, Zhang et al., 2006a). That haem biosynthesis machinery and DMT1 were functionally normal in *hbd* affected mice, strengthens the possibility that Sec15l1 may play a direct role in endosomal vesicle docking and cargo delivery (Zhang et al., 2006a). Given these observations were exclusive to the erythroid cell, the existence of a LIP in other cell types is still to be convincingly challenged, and remains a strong, albeit elusive, intracellular component.

1.2.3.3 Cytosolic Iron Storage

Following transit in the LIP, iron not required for immediate cellular use, is sequestered into the cytosolic iron storage protein, ferritin (Harrison and Arosio, 1996). Storage of iron in ferritin is critical to prevent redox interactions and associated toxicity of the unbound metal (Arosio et al., 2009). When metabolic needs increase, iron can be accessed from this 'reservoir' and transported to sites of utilisation. Ferritin exists as a high molecular weight polymer comprised of heavy (H-ferritin) and light (L-ferritin) chain subunits (Harrison and Arosio, 1996). Assembly of these subunits forms a 12 nm wide protein shell and ~8 nm wide core which is capable of storing > 4500 atoms of iron (Chasteen and Harrison, 1999, Harrison et al., 1974, Iancu, 1992). When iron is sequestered into ferritin, it is oxidised and deposited as ferric oxohydroxide, a concentrated and compact iron mineral (Arosio et al., 2009). This allows iron to be stored in a safe yet soluble and bioavailable form, and accounts for the proteins high iron binding capacity (which is 200 times that of haemoglobin) (Chasteen and Harrison, 1999).

Amino acid sequence identity between H- and L-subunits is ~55%, and the proportion of these subunits is tissue dependent (Arosio et al., 1978). Approximately two thirds of the ferritin in the heart and brain (energy producing organs) is comprised of H-ferritin, whereas 90% of ferritin in the liver and spleen (iron storage organs) is comprised of   L-ferritin (Arosio et al., 1978, Chasteen and Harrison, 1999). This most likely reflects the differing properties of each subunit. Only H-ferritin possesses ferroxidase activity and can oxidise iron (Levi et al., 1988, Santambrogio et al., 1996) and thus, anti-oxidant activity is more pronounced in ferritins which are rich in H-subunits (Arosio et al., 2009). L-ferritin facilitates nucleation of iron for mineralisation, and thus ferritins rich in L-subunits are physically more stable, contain a larger amount of iron in the cavity, and are more suited to long term iron storage (Arosio et al., 2009, Ford et al., 1984, Rucker et al., 1996).

Interestingly, naturally occurring genetic mutations in *H-ferritin* appear rare (Arosio et al., 2009). Only one case has been identified in which mutations in this gene were a causative factor of disease pathology in humans (Cremonesi et al., 2003, Kato et al., 2001). Instead, murine models act to highlight the clinical consequences which could arise from *H-ferritin* mutations. Conditional knockout of *H-ferritin* in the liver, decreases iron storage and induces liver damage (Darshan et al., 2009), and deletion of *H-ferritin* in mice is embryonically lethal (Ferreira et al., 2000). Collectively, these models indicate that the ferroxidase activity of H-ferritin is important for iron storage and also, essential for life and during embryonic development. Genetic variations in *L-ferritin* cause the hereditary neurodegenerative disease, neuroferritinopathy (or hereditary ferritinopathy) (Curtis et al., 2001). Disease pathogenesis is characterised by progressive accumulation of iron largely in the central nervous system, and ensuing oxidative stress which leads to severe neuronal loss, atrophy and cerebellar ataxia (Barbeito et al., 2010, Vidal et al., 2008). Collectively, these findings highlight that both L- and H-ferritin are important for healthy iron metabolism.

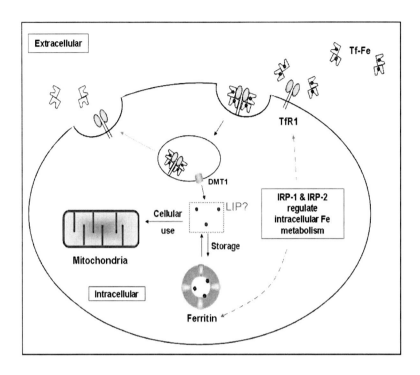

Figure 1.1 Schematic diagram of the physiological pathways of cellular iron uptake and metabolism. Iron (red dot) is transported throughout the serum, bound to the iron transport protein, transferrin (Tf). At the plasma cell membrane, transferrin-bound iron (Tf-Fe) binds to the transferrin receptor 1 (TfR1). Receptor mediated endocytosis internalises the Tf-TfR1 complex, and a decrease in endosomal pH releases iron from the complex for transport out of the endosome to the cytosol by the divalent metal transporter 1 (DMT1). Apo-Tf-TfR1 is recycled back to the cell surface, and Tf is returned to the circulation. Iron is then thought to transiently enter the putative intracellular compartment known as the labile iron pool (LIP). Subsequently, iron that is not required for immediate cellular use, can be stored within the cytosolic storage protein, ferritin. Iron which is required for the metabolic production of iron sulfur clusters and haem, is transported to the mitochondrion for processing. Intracellular iron metabolism is regulated by iron regulatory proteins-1 and -2 (IRP1 and IRP2), which post-transcriptionally control the expression of *TfR1* and *ferritin* in response to cytosolic iron levels.

1.2.4 Mitochondrial Iron Metabolism

Alternatively to the storage of iron within cytosolic ferritin, iron which is required for cellular processes, may be trafficked to sites of iron utilisation, such as the mitochondrion (Sheftel and Lill, 2009). The function of the mitochondrion has traditionally been linked to the provision of energy for the cell, given that they generate approximately 90% of the energy that cells (Kidd, 2005) and accordingly tissues, organs and organisms, need to survive. In addition to its role as an energy powerhouse, the mitochondrion is now appreciated to be crucial for iron metabolism (Napier et al., 2005). Indeed, the mitochondrion is the major site for ISC synthesis (Muhlenhoff and Lill, 2000) and the unique site for haem synthesis (Ponka, 1997). This makes it one of the most active intracellular consumers of iron. That mitochondria have these special requirements for iron, supports the notion that specific mechanisms may exist to target iron to this organelle (Levi and Rovida, 2009, Sheftel et al., 2007, Zhang et al., 2005a). Although we have a good appreciation of mitochondrial iron usage, less is known of such iron trafficking pathways which specifically target iron to the mitochondrion.

1.2.4.1 Mitochondrial Iron Uptake

A number of different mechanisms have been proposed which outline how iron may be transported across mitochondrial membranes, and made available for use in the mitochondrial matrix. As previously discussed, one possibility is that iron could be transferred directly into this organelle *via* endosomal-mitochondrial interactions following the 'kiss and run' hypothesis in co-ordination with Sec15l1 (Sheftel et al., 2007, Zhang et al., 2005a). However, this system has only been identified in erythrocytes

(Sheftel et al., 2007). A second mechanism of mitochondrial iron acquisition, may be *via* the recently identified proteins, mitoferrin1 (Mtfrn1) and mitoferrin2 (Mtfrn2), which are members of the mitochondrial solute carrier family (Paradkar et al., 2009, Shaw et al., 2006). Mtfrn1 is highly expressed in developing erythrocytes (Shaw et al., 2006). Preliminary data indicate that the inner mitochondrial membrane ATP-binding cassette transporter, ABCB10, physically interacts with Mtfrn1 (Chen et al., 2009), and that this association stabilises Mtfrn1 and increases mitochondrial iron import in the developing erythrocyte (Chen et al., 2009, Shaw et al., 2006). In non-erythroid cells, both Mtfrn1 and Mtfrn2 appear to take part in mitochondrial iron uptake (Paradkar et al., 2009). Deletion of Mtfrn1 and Mtfrn2 *in vivo*, impairs mitochondrial iron acquisition by greater than 90%, and decreases haem and ISC synthesis (Paradkar et al., 2009, Shaw et al., 2006, Zhang et al., 2006b). However, the absence of a lethal deleterious phenotype, indicates that the mitochondrion might possess further unidentified methods by which it can take up iron.

1.2.4.2 Mitochondrial Iron Storage

The process of respiration inside the mitochondrion generates high levels of intrinsic ROS (Arosio et al., 2009). This means meticulous pathways must exist to handle iron entering the mitochondrial matrix, and prevent Fenton chemistry with ROS substrates. In some cell types, supply and storage of mitochondrial iron is achieved by the recently identified protein, mitochondrial ferritin (MIT ferritin) (Levi et al., 2001, Santambrogio et al., 2007). Like cytosolic ferritins, MIT ferritin can bind iron and is capable of detoxification due its ferroxidase activity (Campanella et al., 2009, Levi et al., 2001). Additionally, MIT ferritin shares high sequence homology (~80%) and is similar in crystallographic structure to H-ferritin (Langlois d'Estaintot et al., 2004). However, expression of MIT ferritin appears to be limited to cell types with high metabolic activity such as cardiomyocytes and neurons (Santambrogio et al., 2007). Immunoreactive tissue staining recently confirmed, on a visual basis, the presence of MIT ferritin in cells of particularly high mitochondrial density (Snyder et al., 2010). Although MIT ferritin plays a role in mitochondrial iron storage, its expression is lowest, if detectable at all, in hepatocytes and other cell types which are directly involved in iron storage (Santambrogio et al., 2007). This is probably because it serves as an 'aid' for storage of additional iron in cell types which have increased iron demands due to their increased metabolic processes and active respiration (Levi and Rovida, 2009).

No diseases have yet been identified which are caused by mutations in MIT ferritin mutations. In this respect, unlike cytosolic ferritin, MIT ferritin does not appear to be essential for basic cell survival (Levi et al., 2001). However, MIT ferritin has been demonstrated to be of benefit in some pathological situations. For instance, in cells which exhibit a phenotype of mitochondrial iron overload, respiratory deficiencies and oxidative damage, induction of MIT ferritin rescued respiratory function, sequestered iron, and preserved mitochondrial DNA integrity (Campanella et al., 2004). This suggested that MIT ferritin could play a role in sequestering iron to prevent iron related toxicity and ROS generation (Campanella et al., 2004).

1.2.4.3 Iron Sulfur Cluster Synthesis

Depending on metabolic demands, iron that reaches the mitochondrial matrix may also be used in ISC or haem synthetic pathways (Levi et al., 2001). The mitochondrion is the major site of ISC biosynthesis, providing ISCs for mitochondrial, cytosolic and nuclear proteins (Gerber and Lill, 2002). It is here that we see how energy production and mitochondrial iron utilisation are intricately linked. The mitochondrial energy producing pathways of the tricarboxylic acid cycle and electron transport chain, both depend on enzymes with ISC prosthetic groups to function, such as mitochondrial aconitase and respiratory chain complexes I (NADH dehydrogenase) and II (succinate dehydrogenase) (Rouault and Tong, 2008).

The mechanism of ISC biogenesis is a complex process. To date, we have knowledge that over 20 different proteins are involved in eukaryotic ISC formation and maturation (Lill and Muhlenhoff, 2008, Rouault and Tong, 2008). The scope of this encompasses proteins which are involved in initial cluster assembly through to incorporation of clusters in recipient apoproteins of a mitochondrial, cytosolic or nuclear location (Sheftel and Lill, 2009). Briefly, ISCs are assembled on the ISC unit scaffold proteins, Iscu1/2 (Richardson et al., 2010), using sulfur provided by the cysteine desulfurase, Nfs1 (Kispal et al., 1999, Land and Rouault, 1998), and iron that is most likely provided by the inner mitochondrial membrane protein, frataxin (Leidgens et al., 2010, Wang and Craig, 2008, Yoon and Cowan, 2003). Mutations in *FRDA* (which encodes frataxin) cause the severe degenerative disease, Friedreich's ataxia (Campuzano et al., 1996, Puccio et al., 2001). In this disease, loss of frataxin causes mitochondrial iron accumulation and ISC deficiency, and study of this disease provided the first evidence linking frataxin to ISC synthesis (Richardson et al., 2010). Latter studies have found that human frataxin can bind up to six or seven iron ions, form a complex with ISC scaffold proteins, and in an iron-dependent manner, mediate the transfer of iron for ISC formation *in vitro* (Yoon and Cowan, 2003). A direct interaction has also been demonstrated between the yeast ISC assembly protein, Isu1, and the conserved tryptophan in the β-sheet protein structure of the yeast frataxin homologue, Yfh1 (Leidgens et al., 2010, Wang and Craig, 2008).

Release of ISCs from assembly proteins and consequent incorporation into recipient mitochondrial apoproteins, involves a host of additional molecules, (*e.g.,* Ssq1, Jac1, Mge1 and Grx5) (Levi and Rovida, 2009). Clusters with cytosolic recipients must be exported out of the mitochondrion. Although it has not been directly demonstrated, it is thought that the large, inner mitochondrial membrane ATP-binding cassette, ABCB7, may perform this role (Allikmets et al., 1999, Bekri et al., 2000, Cavadini et al., 2007). Deletion of the yeast homologue of *ABCB7*, *Atm1p*, causes mitochondrial iron accumulation and hinders assembly of cytosolic ISC-containing proteins, whilst mitochondrial ISC-containing proteins remain unaffected (Kispal et al., 1999). In human pathology, missense mutations in *ABCB7*, cause mitochondrial iron accumulation and loss of cytosolic ISC proteins in the disease X-linked sideroblastic anaemia with ataxia (Bekri et al., 2000), supporting the possibility that ABCB7 is an ISC export molecule.

1.2.4.4 Haem Synthesis

In addition to the ISC synthetic pathway, the haem synthetic pathway is an equally major consumer of mitochondrial iron. The haem synthetic pathway is in fact exclusive to the mitochondrion (Ponka, 1997). Similarly to ISCs, haem prosthetic groups are essential components of many cellular process, such as haemoglobin and myoglobin, which are used for oxygen transport and oxygen storage, respectively (Sheftel and Lill, 2009). The haem synthetic pathway is well characterised and has been extensively reviewed (Ajioka et al., 2006, Levi and Rovida, 2009, Ponka, 1997, Sheftel and Lill, 2009). For the purpose of my studies herein, it is important to acknowledge the roles of frataxin and ferrochelatase (Fech) in the context of haem biosynthesis.

In the final step of haem synthesis, Fech is responsible for inserting iron into protoporphyrin IX to produce haem (Napier et al., 2005). In the context of disease, this observation is supported by the molecular characteristics of the human inherited disorder, erythropoietic protoporphyria, in which mutations in the gene encoding Fech and deficiencies in Fech enzyme activity can cause increases in iron free protoporphyrin, which is associated with a painful skin photosensitivity (Rüfenacht et al., 1998).

The presence of an ISC moiety in the haem producing protein, Fech, underscores the interdependency of the two major iron consuming pathways of haem and ISC synthesis (Sheftel and Lill, 2009). In addition to its proposed role as an iron donor in ISC synthesis, *in vitro* evidence suggests frataxin also acts as a high-affinity Fech binding partner, capable of mediating the final step in haem synthesis (Yoon and Cowan, 2004). Indeed, frataxin-Fech interactions appear to increase the Fech-catalysed insertion of iron into protoporphyrin IX (Richardson et al., 2010, Yoon and Cowan, 2004). Furthermore, the potential binding site for an iron donor protein (*e.g.,* frataxin) has been revealed from the x-ray crystal structure of Fech (Yoon and Cowan, 2004), and NMR spectroscopy has identified putative interfaces between which Fech and frataxin could bind (He et al., 2004).

Interestingly, recent research has demonstrated that Fech forms an oligomeric complex with both the mitochondrial iron importer, Mtfrn1, and the mitochondrial inner membrane ATP binding cassette protein, ABCB10, in erythroid cells *in vitro* (Chen et al., 2010). Considering the high iron requirements of developing erythrocytes, such a Mtfrn1-ABCB10-Fech complex may represent a unique, efficient and safe mechanism for induction of iron into the haem synthetic pathway in this cell type (Anderson and Vulpe, 2009, Chen et al., 2010).

It is unknown how haem is exported from the mitochondrion to the cytosol. Though members of the ATP-binding cassette super-family such as ABCG2 and ABCB10, or the feline leukemic virus subgroup C receptor, have been identified as possible candidates to perform this function (Jonker et al., 2002, Quigley et al., 2004, Shirihai et al., 2000).

1.3 IRON HOMEOSTASIS

As mentioned, body iron stores must be kept impeccably balanced considering the body has no effective means for excreting iron (McCance and Widdowson, 1938), and that iron deficiency or excess have serious biological ramifications (Murphy and Oudit, 2010, Rouault, 2006, Rouault and Tong, 2008, Thomas and Jankovic, 2004). To ensure dietary iron absorption and body iron stores are kept at levels suffice to meet metabolic requirements, tight and complex regulatory pathways are in place. The intrinsic cellular environment and systemic circulatory system, possess distinct systems by which they co-ordinate iron homeostasis (Hentze et al., 2010), as discussed below.

1.3.1 Cellular Iron Homeostasis

Uptake and storage of intracellular iron is largely controlled by iron regulatory proteins-1 and -2 (IRP1 and IRP2), in coordination with iron-responsive elements (IREs) that are found within transcripts that encode proteins of iron metabolism (Rouault, 2006). The IRP-IRE regulatory system responds to changes in cytosolic iron status, and affords IRP1 and IRP2 post-transcriptional control of cytosolic iron levels to ensure homeostasis is maintained within the intracellular environment (Rouault, 2006) (Figure 1.1).

The stem-loop IRE structure is found in either the 3' or 5' untranslated region (UTR) of mRNA that encodes molecules involved in: (i) iron uptake *e.g. TfR1* and *DMT1* (3' UTR); (ii) iron storage *e.g. H-* and *L-ferritin* (5' UTR); and (iii) iron utilisation *e.g. mitochondrial aconitase* and *5-aminolevinate synthase* (5' UTR) (Galy et al., 2005, Hentze et al., 2010, Wallander et al., 2006, Wingert et al., 2005). In iron deficient cells *in vitro*, IRP-IRE binding acts to stabilise or repress mRNA translation, depending on IRE location in either the 3' or 5' UTR (Hentze et al., 2010). In this manner, IRP binding at the 3' UTR of *TfR1*, protects the transcript from degradation, whereas binding at the 5' UTR within IREs of *H-* and *L-ferritin*, interferes with translational initiation (Hentze and Kuhn, 1996, Rouault and Klausner, 1997, Schneider et al., 1994, Wallander et al., 2006). Thus, IRPs orchestrate the cellular response to iron depletion by increasing cellular iron uptake *via* TfR1, and decreasing cellular cytosolic iron storage within H- and L-ferritin, as a mechanism to re-equilibrate cytosolic iron levels (Hentze and Kuhn, 1996, Rouault and Klausner, 1997, Schneider et al., 1994, Wallander et al., 2006). In cells that are iron replete, IRPs do not bind to IREs (Rouault, 2006). This allows ferritin and other transcripts which have an IRE in the 5' UTR to be freely translated, while the TfR1 transcript is cleaved and consequently degraded (Rouault, 2006).

Although IRP1 and IRP2 share high sequence homology (Rouault et al., 1990, Samaniego et al., 1994, Galy et al., 2008, Meyron-Holtz et al., 2004b), they sense cytosolic iron levels by different mechanisms (Galy et al., 2008, Meyron-Holtz et al., 2004b). IRP1 is a bifunctional protein, and its mRNA-binding activity is determined by the presence of an ISC (Kuhn and Hentze, 1992, Theil and Eisenstein, 2000). In iron-replete cells, the presence of an ISC cluster in IRP1, enables IRP1 to function as a cytosolic aconitase (Hentze et al., 2010), and prevents IRP1-IRE binding (Kwok and Richardson, 2002). Whereas in iron-deplete cells, IRP1 apo-protein binds IREs with high affinity (Rouault, 2006). Unlike IRP1, IRP2 does not contain an ISC cluster (Richardson and Ponka, 1997). Rather, in iron-replete cells, IRP2 is rapidly degraded by a proteasome-dependent mechanism (Richardson and Ponka, 1997).

The differing mechanisms by which IRP1 and IRP2 act, raises the possibility that these two proteins may have distinct functions (Galy et al., 2008). Initially, *in vitro* evidence derived from a breadth of cell lines, indicated that IRP1 was the predominant mammalian regulator of post-transcriptional iron metabolism, though more recently, *in vivo* experiments have contradicted this (Galy et al., 2008, Meyron-Holtz et al., 2004a, Meyron-Holtz et al., 2004b). Constitutive inactivation of both *IRP1* and *IRP2* causes embryonic lethality *in vivo* (Smith et al., 2006), and underscores that the IRP-IRE system is a necessity for cellular viability. But individual knockout models show that deletion of *IRP1* alone does not compromise iron metabolism, as IRP2 was able to maintain iron homeostasis in its place (Meyron-Holtz et al., 2004a). However, deletion of *IRP2* alone, significantly misregulates iron metabolism and causes neurodegeneration in mice, most likely because IRP1 was not able to compensate for the loss of IRP2 (Meyron-Holtz et al., 2004a). Studies indicate that while IRP1 contributes to basal iron metabolism, IRP2 dominates post-transcriptional regulation of iron metabolism *in vivo* and at physiological oxygen tension (Meyron-Holtz et al., 2004a, Meyron-Holtz et al., 2004b).

1.3.2 Systemic Iron Homeostasis

Recent research has identified a number of new molecules which are now understood to be key regulators of systemic iron levels. Of central importance is the anti-microbial peptide, hepcidin, that was first identified in human serum (Krause et al., 2000) and urine (Park et al., 2001) at the turn of the 21st century. Hepcidin is predominantly synthesised in the liver, initially as an 84 amino acid precursor protein that is encoded by the human hepcidin gene, *HAMP* (Lee and Beutler, 2009). Post-translational cleavage is inferred to produce the biologically active 25 amino acid form, which is secreted into the serum to systemically regulate the equilibrium of iron (Park et al., 2001, Pigeon et al., 2001, Valore and Ganz, 2008, Wallace et al., 2006). In addition to the liver, hepcidin expression has also been identified in the heart, albeit at much lower levels (Merle et al., 2007). Little is known about the putative role of hepcidin in the heart. However, initial studies suggest that myocardial hepcidin may have a local, rather than systemic effect, most likely in the cardioprotection against disease and infection (Merle et al., 2007).

Hepatocyte secreted hepcidin co-ordinates circulating serum iron levels *via* interactions with the iron export molecule, ferroportin1 (Lee and Beutler, 2009). In response to appropriate stimuli such as high iron levels or those mentioned below, hepcidin binds to ferroportin1 on the cell surface,

27

causing ferroportin1 to be internalised and subsequently degraded by the lysosome (Nemeth et al., 2006, Nemeth et al., 2004). Loss of ferroportin1 by this mechanism causes intracellular iron retention and regulates the entry of iron into the serum from major iron-releasing cells such as macrophages, hepatocytes and intestinal enterocytes (Knutson et al., 2005, Knutson et al., 2003, Nemeth et al., 2004).

The complete systemic iron regulatory story has not yet been comprehensively elucidated. A number of converging systemic stimuli, which act *via* hepatocyte cell surface proteins (*e.g.* hemojuvelin), appear to influence hepatic hepcidin expression (Hentze et al., 2010). Hepatocyte cell surface proteins in turn, activate cell signal transduction pathways within the hepatocyte to alter transcription of *HAMP* (Darshan and Anderson, 2009). Notable regulatory influences on hepcidin include: (i) erythropoetic signals; (ii) inflammation and infection; (iii) hypoxia; and importantly (iv) systemic iron levels (Ganz and Nemeth, 2006, Hentze et al., 2010, Peyssonnaux et al., 2007, Truksa et al., 2007, Verga Falzacappa et al., 2007, Wrighting and Andrews, 2006). Indeed, hepcidin expression is enhanced by dietary or parenteral iron loading, as a negative feedback loop to prevent further intestinal iron absorption (Hentze et al., 2010, Pigeon et al., 2001). The precise mechanism by which hepatocytes directly sense iron to regulate hepcidin expression, is a continuing point of research.

1.4 IRON IN DISEASE

The array of diseases and pathological phenotypes caused by imbalances in iron indeed underscore the importance of healthy iron metabolism and homeostasis. As mentioned, the ability of iron to cycle between its two stable oxidation states, facilitates mandatory metabolic functions, *via* electron exchange (Kalinowski and Richardson, 2005). However, this quality also enables iron to cause harm by way of oxidative stress.

Regular oxygen metabolism generates an assortment of by-products. These include ROS such as superoxide ($O_2^{\cdot-}$), hydroxyl (OH$^{\cdot}$), nitric oxide (NO$^{\cdot}$), peroxynitrite (ONOO^{-}) and hydrogen peroxide (H_2O_2) (Kalinowski and Richardson, 2005). ROS are highly reactive and potentially damaging to biomolecules. However, at low concentrations, they can act as second messengers, gene regulators and/or mediators of cellular activation (Polla, 1999) To control and balance the production of ROS, cells posses a set of anti-oxidant and detoxifying enzymes such as superoxide dismutase, catalase and glutathione, that to an extent, can manage free radical generation. An imbalance between ROS production and anti-oxidant defence, for example during iron overload, induces a state of 'oxidative stress', in which ROS interact with proteins, lipids and DNA, causing their dysfunction, and ultimately, cell death (Barnham et al., 2004) The brain is at heightened risk from oxidative damage, considering its high oxygen consumption (which represents 20% of total body basal O_2 consumption), abundance of iron, relatively lower levels of anti-oxidants, and tendency to accumulate metals (Gaeta and Hider, 2005).

An oxidative stress hypothesis has been suggested to be at least in part, responsible for the pathological degeneration observed in many neurodegenerative disorders, such as Alzheimer's disease, Parkinson's disease and Friedreich's ataxia, as described below. For the most part, iron is thought to play a central role in the mediation of such oxidative stress. However, it is not yet known whether this role is as a primary causal agent, or as a secondary mediator of disease progression.

1.4.1 Alzheimer's Disease

Alzheimer's disease (AD) is the most common age-related neurodegenerative disorder, and is characterized by the progressive loss of cognitive and behavioural functions that are associated with the temporal and frontal lobes of the brain (Bush and Tanzi, 2002). The presence of toxic amyloid-β aggregates in extracellular senile plaques and loss of cortical neurons are defining pathological hallmarks of AD (Honda et al., 2004). Several lines of evidence suggest that iron dyshomeostasis and iron-induced oxidative stress play a role in AD neurodegeneration. Changes in the levels of iron, ferritin and Tf have been reported in the hippocampus and cerebral cortex of the AD brain, which represent key centres of memory and thought processing that are lost in the clinical profile of this disease (Honda et al., 2005, Sipe et al., 2002). Furthermore, in areas of particular neurodegeneration, iron has been shown to accumulate at a faster pace than ferritin production (Connor et al., 1992), and significant associations between unbound, redox-active iron and the presence of amyloid-β senile plaques have been demonstrated (Smith et al., 1997).

Additionally, the identification of an aberrant IRE (IRE-type II) in the 5' UTR region of *amyloid precursor protein* (APP) mRNA may further support the connection between iron metabolism and AD (Rogers et al., 2002). APP is an integral membrane protein which is cleaved by β-secretase to generate amyloid-β. In the presence of iron, *amyloid precursor protein* translation is up-regulated, promoting increased cleavage and deposition of amyloid-β fragments (Atwood et al., 1999), which aggregate to form plaques. Significantly, in response to intracellular iron chelation, *amyloid precursor protein* 5' UTR translation can be down-regulated through mediation of IRE-IRP binding (Rogers et al., 2002). However, this novel IRE is somewhat uncharacteristic of typical IREs that mediate regulation of genes by iron (Hentze and Kuhn, 1996, Richardson and Ponka, 1997). As such, further research is required to positively confirm these observations and to confirm the functional activity of the IRE in amyloid precursor protein.

1.4.2 Parkinson's Disease

Parkinson's disease (PD) is the next most common neurodegenerative disorder to AD (Levenson, 2003). In PD, cumulative loss of dopaminergic neurons in the substantia nigra pars compacta, results in decreased dopamine production, and gives rise to the characteristic dysregulation of bodily movement evident in PD patients (Levenson, 2003). Notably, increased iron concentrations have been observed in the dopaminergic neurons of PD patients (Levenson, 2003). Furthermore, MRI studies indicate that the level of iron which has accumulated within these neurons, is related to the severity of PD symptoms (Bartzokis et al., 1997, Gorell et al., 1995, Ryvlin et al., 1995). A consistent histopathological finding in PD is the aggregation of α-synuclein into Lewy bodies (el-Agnaf and Irvine, 2002). It has been suggested that iron-catalysed oxidative reactions, convert α-synuclein from its inert α-helical form, into the β-pleated sheet conformation seen in Lewy bodies (el-Agnaf and Irvine, 2002). Toxicity induced by α-synuclein in the presence of iron results in apoptotic mechanisms which are thought to be partly responsible for dopaminergic neuronal cell death in this disease (el-Agnaf and Irvine, 2002).

Although current findings propose a role for iron in neurodegeneration, it is not known whether its function is as a primary or secondary agonist (Zecca et al., 2004). Several studies have provided evidence that ferritin and the brain iron binding protein, neuromelanin, fail to attenuate iron in a safe and inert form in PD. For instance, similar to the situation in AD, it has been suggested that iron accumulation outweighs ferritin production in PD (Faucheux et al., 2002, Thompson et al., 2003). The studies of Faucheux *et. al.* suggest that stagnate IRP1-RNA binding activity in the substantia nigra of PD patients could explain the lack of up-regulation in ferritin expression in response to increased nigral iron levels (Faucheux et al., 2002). There is also a possibility that iron bound to neuromelanin may remain redox active. A significant increase in the redox activity of neuromelanin aggregates has been observed in PD patients compared to control subjects, with highest levels reported in patients with the most severe neuronal loss (Faucheux et al., 2003).

1.4.3 Friedreich's Ataxia

Friedreich's ataxia (FA) is the most common form of inherited autosomal ataxia (Campuzano et al., 1996, Gakh et al., 2006, Koutnikova et al., 1997). Onset of symptoms occurs in adolescence, with patient life expectancy averaging 36 years from the time of onset (De Michele et al., 1996). Clinical features include progressive degeneration of the large sensory neurons and spinocerebellar tracts, and the development of a severe cardiomyopathy (Durr et al., 1996, Harding, 1981). Neuronal degeneration of cerebral motor cortex areas and dorsal root ganglia account for most neurological symptoms (Cossee et al., 2000), while cardiac hypertrophy is the primary cause of premature death in patients (Alper and Narayanan, 2003, Bradley et al., 2000, Delatycki et al., 2000).

In the majority of cases, the molecular genetic defect in FA involves trinucleotide $(GAA)_n$ repeat hyperexpansions within intron one (chromosome 9q13) of the gene, *FRDA* (Campuzano et al., 1996, Durr et al., 1996) in which frataxin is encoded (Campuzano et al., 1996, Lodi et al., 2002). As a consequence, transcription is impaired and *FRDA* gene expression is decreased, accounting for a decrease in frataxin protein levels to below 30% of normal (Van Driest et al., 2005).

Although the precise function of frataxin has not been defined, strong evidence has accumulated that indicates it plays a role in mitochondrial iron metabolism (Babcock et al., 1997, Bradley et al., 2000, Campuzano et al., 1997, Foury and Cazzalini, 1997, Radisky et al., 1999, Wong et al., 1999), and most notably ISC and haem synthetic pathways (as discussed in Sections 1.2.4.3 and 1.2.4.4, respectively). Studies using yeast cells demonstrated that deletion of the frataxin yeast homologue, *Yfh1*, resulted in an accumulation of mitochondrial iron (Babcock et al., 1997, Foury and Cazzalini, 1997, Rötig et al., 1997). This is supported by observations of accumulated iron within myocardial mitochondria of FA patients upon post-mortem examination (Lamarche et al., 1993, Wong et al., 1999), and also in the mitochondrion of cardiomyocytes from muscle creatine kinase (MCK) frataxin knockout mice (Figure 1.2) (Puccio et al., 2001).

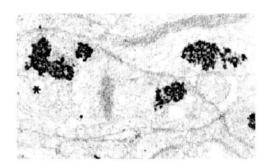

Figure 1.2 Iron accumulation in Friedreich's ataxia. Transmission electron micrograph showing the presence of black iron deposits in the mitochondrion of cardiomyocytes in the muscle creatine kinase (MCK) conditional frataxin knockout mouse model. Adapted from Puccio et. al., 2001.

As mentioned (Sections 1.2.3.4 and 1.2.4.4), experimental observations suggest frataxin plays a role in mitochondrial iron trafficking (Napier et al., 2005). Evidence of decreased activity of ISC-dependent mitochondrial respiratory chain cytochrome complexes and also aconitase activity in FA patients, are testament to the involvement of frataxin in mitochondrial metabolism (Rötig et al., 1997). In addition, frataxin has been suggested to possess ferroxidation and mineralisation activities that enable it to detoxify surplus iron, limiting iron-induced oxidative damage (Gakh et al., 2006, O'Neill et al., 2005, Park et al., 2003, Park et al., 2002). However, further studies are still required to definitively assess the precise function of frataxin and its role in mitochondrial iron metabolism (Napier et al., 2005).

A long standing hypothesis is that FA results from iron-mediated oxidative stress. Without effective chelation, free iron in FA fibroblasts participate in reactions with superoxide generated within the mitochondrion to produce ROS (Wong et al., 1999). Mitochondrial DNA may be particularly affected by ROS, given that it lacks the protection of histone proteins found in nuclear DNA (Eaton and Qian, 2002). Furthermore, ISC proteins (such as respiratory chain enzymes) are exquisitely sensitive to ROS (Wong et al., 1999), and thus ROS may destabilise complexes of the respiratory chain, adding to the amplifying cycle of oxidative damage suggested to occur in FA (Bradley et al., 2000, Eaton and Qian, 2002).

Recent observations challenge the hypothesis that oxidative stress is involved in the pathogenesis of FA, as some frataxin mouse models lack measurable quantities of oxidative stress markers (Seznec et al., 2004, Seznec et al., 2005). Complementing this observation, attempts to reduce disease severity by administration of the mitochondrial anti-oxidant, MnTBAP, had no effect on the survival rates of frataxin knockout mice (Seznec et al., 2005). These reports suggest that free radical production is only a minor component of FA pathophysiology, at least in mouse models of FA. Increased levels of 8-hydroxy-2'-deoxyguanosine (an oxidative stress marker) (Schulz et al., 2000) have been observed in patients, and correlations between the severity of lipid peroxidation and the duration and severity of this disease in patients (Bradley et al., 2004) suggests that oxidative stress is still an important consideration in the human disease.

1.5 IRON CHELATORS FOR THE TREATMENT DISEASE

The accumulation of iron at sites of neuronal degeneration in AD and PD, and within mitochondria of degenerated cardiomyocytes in FA, demonstrate the toxicity that can arise when tissues accrue excess iron in disease. Furthermore, they also necessitate the development of therapeutic agents that are able to target and remove iron.

Iron chelation therapy involves the use of ligating drugs that avidly bind iron from biological systems. The idea of targeted iron removal is not in fact, a new concept. Iron chelators have been employed to treat conditions of iron overload such as β-Thalassemia since the 1960s (Chaston and Richardson, 2003b, Kalinowski and Richardson, 2005). However, it is only more recently that their roles in other diseases such as neurodegeneration and cancer (discussed in Section 1.5.1, below) have been considered (Richardson et al., 2001, Chaston and Richardson, 2003b, Kalinowski and Richardson, 2005).

1.5.1 Iron Chelation for the Treatment of Cancer

Iron chelation therapy was initially designed to alleviate the toxic effects of excess iron in diseases of iron overload and accumulation (Kalinowski 2007 Chem research in toxicology). However, the more recently recognised iron-requiring properties of neoplastic cells, has stimulated research into the design and synthesis of iron chelators for the treatment of cancer. Indeed, metabolic inhibitors represent an important class of anti-tumour agents, and in the past, medicinal chemists have targeted the nutrient folate for the development of anti-cancer therapies (Richardson et al., 2009). This was based on the rapid replication of neoplastic cells, and the critical need for folate in DNA synthesis (Richardson et al., 2009). Indeed, folate-targeting agents such as methotrexate have been commercial successful and are a mainstay in the treatment of many neoplastic disorders (McGuire, 2003).

Like folate, iron is also now understood to be critical for neoplastic cell growth, due to the rapid rate of neoplastic cell replication, and the critical requirement for iron during DNA synthesis (Richardson et al., 2009). As mentioned (Section 1.1), during the rate-limiting step of DNA synthesis, iron is required in the active site of the enzyme, ribonucleotide reductase (Thelander and Reichard, 1979), and on this premise, the targeted removal of iron from neoplastic cells *via* the use of iron chelators, could inhibit their rate of replication. Neoplastic cells also have increased expression of the iron uptake molecule, TfR1 (Sutherland et al., 1981, Taetle and Honeysett, 1987, Trowbridge and Lopez, 1982), and treatment with monoclonal anti-TfR1 antibody has been demonstrated to inhibit human tumour cell growth *in vitro* (Trowbridge and Lopez, 1982). Likewise, increased expression of the iron storage molecule, ferritin, has also been detected in neoplastic tissues compared to normal tissue (Vaughn et al., 1987). These molecular changes in iron metabolism proteins, underscore the high iron requirements of cancer cells, and supports the use of iron chelators as chemotherapeutic agents.

1.5.2 Properties to be Considered in the Design of Clinically Useful Iron Chelators

When designing any new therapeutic agent for clinical application, the onus is on developing compounds which take maximum effect, while having minimal toxicity to normal physiological processes. For the treatment of iron overload disease, this specifically means designing compounds which bind iron to form a non-toxic metal complex, thus preventing iron from participating in redox activity (Chaston and Richardson, 2003b). Though in the development of iron chelators for the treatment of cancer, iron chelators that are able to redox cycle after binding iron within the neoplastic cell, may be potentially advantageous in damaging the tumour itself (Kalinowski and Richardson, 2007). In designing a clinically successful chelator, a number of factors must be critically considered, as below.

Chelating agents can be designed for either the iron(III) or iron(II) oxidative states, based upon the donor atoms of the ligand (Chaston and Richardson, 2003b, Kalinowski and Richardson, 2005). Chelators that prefer iron(II) contain "soft" donor atoms such as nitrogen and sulfur (Kalinowski and Richardson, 2005). As a consequence of their selectivity for iron(II) over iron(III), iron(II) chelators retain a relatively high affinity for other biologically important divalent metals such as copper(II) and zinc(II) (Liu and Hider, 2002). Hence, such ligands may inhibit the activity of metallo-enzymes that make use of copper and zinc as co-factors (Liu and Hider, 2002). The major synthetic focus has been on the design of iron(III)-selective chelators which feature "hard" oxygen donor atoms (Chaston and Richardson, 2003b, Kalinowski and Richardson, 2005). Iron(III) chelators are generally more selective for trivalent metal cations over divalent cations. Importantly, unlike divalent metals, most trivalent metals such as aluminium(III) and gallium(III) are not essential for living cells, and hence, iron(III) chelators may be potentially less toxic (Liu and Hider, 2002). Additionally, under aerobic conditions, high-affinity iron(III) chelators, chelate iron(II) to facilitate autoxidation to iron(III) (Chaston and Richardson, 2003b, Harris and Aisen, 1973). As a consequence, high-affinity iron(III)-selective compounds will beneficially bind both iron(III) and iron(II) under most physiological conditions (Chaston and Richardson, 2003b, Liu and Hider, 2002).

A further consideration in the design of any clinically useful agent, is its ability to reach target sites at a sufficient concentration so as to exert its pharmacological effect. In considering this, two facets of chelator design must be considered, namely: (i) route of administration; and (ii) the location of iron intended to be removed. Patient compliance is a major factor impacting treatment success, and hence the route of administration should represent the least invasive method of drug delivery, such as oral administration (Cook, 2007). In order to achieve efficient oral absorption, a chelator should possess appreciable lipid solubility (log $P_{water/octanol}$ > -0.7) (Kalinowski and Richardson, 2005, Liu and Hider, 2002). Lipophilicity not only facilitates penetration *via* the gastrointestinal tract (Tillbrook and Hider, 1998), it is one of three major factors which influence the ability of a chelator to permeate biological membranes such as the blood brain barrier and inner mitochondrial membrane. Penetration of both the gastrointestinal tract (Hollander et al., 1988) and blood brain barrier (Oldendorf, 1974) is also governed by molecular size. To effect > 70% oral absorption, Maxton and colleagues recommend the molecular weight of a chelator be < 500 Daltons (Maxton et al., 1986). Finally, permeability is additionally influenced by ionic state of the chelator, with uncharged, neutral chelators being able to penetrate cell membranes more rapidly than charged molecules (Richardson et al., 1990b, Florence and Attwood, 1988).

In summary, careful consideration is required when investigating new chelators. A compound suitable for the treatment of disease should possess a number of qualities, namely; (i) strong affinity for iron; (ii) low molecular weight; (iii) lipophilicity high enough to accommodate permeation of cell membranes and access to relevant iron stores; (iv) oral activity; and (v) minimal toxicity to normal physiological processes. Taking these factors into consideration, the chelators desferrioxamine and pyridoxal isonicotinoyl hyrdrazone (discussed below) represent two compounds which have been previously investigated for their iron chelating properties.

1.5.3 Desferrioxamine

For three decades, the hexadentate siderophore, desferrioxamine (DFO), has been the only approved iron chelator for human use (Cunningham and Nathan, 2005). DFO possesses an extremely high and specific affinity for iron, binding iron in a 1:1 molar ratio as to co-ordinately saturate the metal ion, minimising the potential of the complex to redox cycle (Kalinowski and Richardson, 2005). Consequently, DFO is able to significantly decrease the oxidative stress in iron-overloaded cells and alleviate symptoms associated with iron-overload disease (Chaston and Richardson, 2003b, Olivieri and Brittenham, 1997). Traditionally, DFO has been employed in the treatment of β-thalassemia to minimise the iron-overload associated with chronic red blood cell transfusions (Chaston and Richardson, 2003b, Olivieri and Brittenham, 1997). Indeed, improvements observed in the survival and well-being of β-thalassemia patients treated with DFO, validates the use of iron chelation therapy in other diseases of iron accumulation and overload (Kalinowski and Richardson, 2005).

Previous studies and clinical trials have also demonstrated the therapeutic benefit of DFO in the treatment of cancer. For example, after a 72 hour exposure to DFO *in vitro*, a > 80% reduction in cell viability was observed in a neuroblastoma cell line (Blatt and Stitely, 1987). Furthermore, in clinical trial, treatment of neuroblastoma patients with 150 mg/kg of DFO over a 5 day period, successfully reduced bone marrow infiltration and tumour size, without causing any significant side effects (Donfrancesco et al., 1990).

However, a number of disadvantages limit the therapeutic use of DFO. Firstly, the highly hydrophilic nature of DFO limits its absorption across the gastrointestinal tract, and its rapid drug metabolism leads to a short plasma half-life (12 minutes) (Aouad et al., 2002, Olivieri and Brittenham, 1997). As a result, parenteral administration is the only option, and involves long subcutaneous infusions from 8 to 12 hours, five to seven times per week (Olivieri and Brittenham, 1997). This, together with the high cost and pain experienced by some patients at the site of injection, have led to a history of poor patient compliance to DFO (Olivieri and Brittenham, 1997, Wong et al., 2004). (Olivieri and Brittenham, 1997, Wong et al., 2004)

1.5.4 Pyridoxal isonicotinoyl hydrazone

The treatment of FA in particular, requires a strategically different approach to that of other neurodegenerative diseases. In addition to blood brain barrier access, chelators must be able to permeate the inner- and outer-mitochondrial membranes to access accumulated iron within cardiomyocytes. Given that cardiac failure is the leading cause of death in FA patients (Delatycki et al., 2000), the development of lipophilic chelators that could fulfil the aforementioned role is critical.

Over twenty years ago, it was shown that the hydrophobic chelator, pyridoxal isonicotinoyl hydrazone (PIH), could permeate the mitochondrion to bind accumulated non-heme iron in rabbit reticulocytes (reticulocyte iron-loaded mitochondrion model) (Ponka et al., 1979a, Richardson et al., 2001). As a possible model chelator for FA treatment, PIH possesses many advantageous characteristics, including: (i) an ability to permeate mitochondrial membranes and bind intra-mitochondrial iron accumulations *in vitro* (Ponka et al., 1979a, Richardson et al., 2001); (ii) oral effectiveness in animals and humans (Brittenham, 1990, Hoy et al., 1979); (iii) high affinity and selectivity for iron over other important

41

biologically relevant metal ions (Richardson et al., 1989); (iv) uncharged state at neutral pH values (*e.g.*, 7.4), facilitating permeation of biological membranes (Richardson et al., 1990a); (v) near optimal lipophilic/hydrophilic balance of the apochelator and iron complex, allowing passage into and out of cells (Ponka et al., 1994); (vi) economical and simple synthesis which involves a one-step Schiff base condensation (Johnson et al., 1982, Ponka et al., 1994); (vii) low cytotoxicity and poor ability to inhibit proliferation and DNA synthesis that is less than that of DFO (Becker and Richardson, 1999, Richardson et al., 1995); and (viii) high iron chelation efficacy both *in vitro* in cultured cells, *in vivo* in animal models and in a clinical trial (Hoy et al., 1979, Ponka et al., 1979b, Richardson et al., 2001, Richardson et al., 1995).

1.6 SPECIFIC OBJECTIVES

Considering the number of people affected by cancer, and the development of multi-drug resistance to current chemotherapeutics, novel agents must be designed for the treatment of cancer. The high metabolic activity of neoplastic cells and hence, their increased need for iron compared to the normal counterparts, validates iron chelation therapy as a potentially useful new therapeutic avenue to explore. Hence, this project aimed to:

1A: Investigate the *in vitro* anti-proliferative activity of the novel DpT and PKIH series of iron chelators, and

1B: Test the *in vivo* anti-tumour activity and impact on metabolic processes of the most potent chelator identified from studies in Objective 1A.

Cardiomyopathy is the leading cause of death in Friedreich's ataxia, and given the toxic mitochondrial iron accumulations observed cardiomyocytes

42

in this disease, iron chelation therapy should likewise be explored as a therapeutic avenue for this disease. Furthermore, little is known regarding the mechanism of mitochondrial iron overload in Friedreich's ataxia. Considering these issues, the current project also aimed to:

2A: Investigate the use of PIH in combination with DFO for the treatment of the severe cardiomyopathy in the MCK mouse model of FA, and

2B: Identify the mechanism of mitochondrial iron loading in the MCK mouse model of FA.

The precise form of iron that accumulates within the mitochondrion of the FA heart has not been successfully elucidated. Furthermore, during the tenure of my thesis, the presence of a cytosolic iron deficiency (in addition to mitochondrial iron overload) in the MCK mouse model of FA became apparent. Given these observations, this project also aimed to:

3A: Explore the ability of iron supplementation to reconstitute the iron deficient cytosol in the MCK mouse model of FA, and

3B: Elucidate the form of iron accumulating within the heart of the MCK mouse model of FA.

CHAPTER 2
MATERIALS AND METHODS

2.1 REAGENTS

2.1.1 Chemicals

Agarose, glacial acetic acid, sodium dodecyl sulfate (SDS) and tris(hydroxymethyl)aminomethane (tris) were purchased from Amresco (Solon, USA). Chloroform, disodium ethylenediaminetetraacetic acid (EDTA), dithiothreitol, ethidium bromide (EtBr), ethylene glycol-bis(2-aminoethylether)-N,N,N',N'-tetraacetic acid (EGTA), glutaraldehyde, magnesium chloride ($MgCl_2$), HEPES, isopropanol, paraformaldehyde, sodium chloride (NaCl), sodium fluoride (NaF), sucrose, tris-HCl and triton X-100 were purchased from Sigma-Aldrich (Sydney, Australia). Glycerol, hydrochloric acid (HCl) and potassium chloride (KCl) were obtained from BDH laboratory supplies. (Biolab, Auckland, New Zealand). Complete protease inhibitors® were obtained from Roche Diagnostics (Mannheim, Germany) and deoxynucleotide triphosphates (dNTPs) from Promega (Sydney, Australia). Phosphate buffered saline (PBS) was from Invitrogen (Melbourne, Australia).

2.1.2 Buffers and Solutions

All buffers and solutions were prepared with de-ionised water. Additionally, diethylpyrocarbonate (DEPC; Sigma-Aldrich)-treated water was used in the preparation of buffers and solutions for RNA analysis. DEPC-treated water was prepared at 0.1% and left overnight. The following day the water was autoclaved at least four times to ensure complete removal of DEPC.

Formulations for general use buffers are as follows: tris-acetate EDTA buffer (TAE; for 20x stock 800 mM tris, 2.2% glacial acetic acid, 100 mM EDTA), and tris-buffered saline (TBS; for 20x stock 25 mM tris, 2.75 mM NaCl, pH 7.6).

For *in vivo* chelator injections, a preparation of sterile vehicle solution was prepared using 15-20% 1,2-propanediol (propylene-glycol; Sigma-Aldrich) made up in 0.9% physiological saline (Baxter Healthcare, Old Toongabbie, Australia).

2.1.3 Diferric-Transferrin

To generate diferric-transferrin (Fe-Tf), human apo-transferrin (Sigma-Aldrich) was labelled with ^{56}Fe (Sigma-Aldrich) or ^{59}Fe (PerkinElmer, Melbourne, Australia) as 0.1M ferric chloride in HCl, as described previously (Richardson and Baker, 1990). The protein concentration and Fe-binding site saturation were assessed using UV-Vis spectrophotometry on a UV-1800 spectrophotometer (Shimadzu Scientific Instruments, Columbia, USA) at absorbances of 280 nm and 465 nm, respectively. In all experiments, fully saturated Fe-Tf was used.

2.2 ANIMALS

2.2.1 Monitoring and Ethics

Experimental mice were used in accordance with the ethical requirements of the University of Sydney. All mice were housed under a 12 h light-dark cycle and fed routinely with basal rodent chow (0.02% iron/kg) and watered *ad libitum*. The general health, behaviour and condition of the mice were monitored daily and body weight recorded twice weekly.

2.2.2 Necroscopy

At the conclusion of experiments mice were weighed, anaesthetised with isofluorane (Abbott Australasia Pty Ltd, Sydney, Australia) and in some instances, blood collected by cardiac puncture. Mice were then sacrificed by cervical dislocation. Organs were removed, weighed and processed accordingly for further analysis (*i.e.,* tissue iron estimation, histological examination, RNA or protein isolation, IRP-RNA binding activity *e.t.c*).

2.3 ANALYSIS OF BIOLOGICAL ANIMAL PARAMETERS

2.3.1 Haematological Indices

Blood taken from anaesthetised mice *via* cardiac puncture was added to haematology tubes containing the anti-coagulant, K^+EDTA (BD Biosciences, Sydney, Australia). Red blood cell (RBC), white blood cell (WBC), haemoglobin (Hb), haematocrit (Hct) and platelet counts were performed using a using a Sysmex K-4500 analyser (TOA Medical Electronics, Kobe, Japan).

2.3.2 Tissue Iron Estimation

To determine tissue non-haem iron concentrations, tissues were acid digested and the samples analysed using inductively coupled plasma atomic emission spectrometry (ICP-AES) at the Bioanalytical Mass Spectrometry Facility (University of New South Wales, Sydney, Australia).

Organs harvested from euthanased mice were rinsed in PBS to remove excess blood. Tissues were then placed in sterile tubes and allowed to dehydrate fully at 55 °C for at least three days in a non humidified incubator. The dry weight of each tissue was then weighed to four decimal places and the tissue placed into a 10 mL glass volumetric flask that had been washed in de-ionised water 4 times then dried. To the volumetric flask, 1 mL of BDH AnalaR® grade nitric acid HNO_3 (Biolab, Auckland, New Zealand) was added and tissues digested overnight at room temperature. The following day, tissues were further digested for 3 h at approximately 90 °C. The solution was allowed to cool for 20 min before 0.4 mL of BDH AnalaR® grade H_2O_2 (Biolab) was added and the solution heated for a further 2 h. The solution was again allowed to cool, and de-ionised water added to a final volume of 10 mL. The solution was then transferred to tubes for ICP-AES assessment. The presence of elemental iron in the glassware, plastic tubes and liquids was corrected for by the preparation of blanks containing all additions apart from tissue. As a control for the accuracy of the ICP-AES, standards were prepared from bovine liver reference material (National Institute of Standards and Technology, Gaithersburg, USA) treated in the same way as the dried mouse tissues. The amount of elemental iron was calculated as µg or mg iron/g of dried tissue.

2.3.3 Histology

Organs harvested from euthanased mice were fixed in 10% neutral buffered formalin (Fronine, Sydney, Australia). Paraffin embedded sections were kindly prepared and stained with hematoxylin and eosin, Gomori-Trichrome or Prussian blue, by Ms Elaine Chew (Faculty of Veterinary Science, University of Sydney, Sydney, Australia). Stained sections were examined and images captured using an Olympus BX51 microscope coupled with a CC-12 camera and analySIS FIVE soft imaging system (Olympus, Sydney, Australia).

2.4 DETECTION OF mRNA USING RT-PCR

2.4.1 Isolation of RNA from Animal Tissues

Standard procedures were used to isolate total RNA from animal tissues (Le and Richardson, 2004). Briefly, tissue samples were homogenised with DEPC-treated tissue grinders in a 1 mL volume of TRIzol® Reagent (Invitrogen). Homogenised tissue samples were incubated at room temperature for 5 min, then 0.2 mL of chloroform was added and the samples shaken vigorously. Samples were incubated for an additional 3 min, centrifuged at 12 000 rpm for 15 min at 4 °C and the aqueous phase transferred to a 0.5 mL volume of isopropanol. After a final 10 min incubation, the samples were centrifuged for 10 min, the supernatant removed and the RNA pellet washed in 75% RNA-grade EtOH (Sigma-Aldrich). RNA pellets were resuspended in DEPC-treated water and concentrations determined by UV-Vis spectrophotometry at 260 nm using a UV-1800 spectrophotometer (Shimadzu Scientific Instruments). The quality of the RNA was also assessed by 1.5% formaldehyde gel electrophoresis and the bands visualised by EtBr staining.

2.4.2 Reverse Transcriptase-Polymerase Chain Reaction

Isolated total RNA was used to perform reverse transcriptase polymerase chain reaction (RT-PCR) by standard procedures (Le and Richardson, 2004). RT-PCR was shown to be semiquantitative by an optimisation protocol, which demonstrated that it was in the log phase of amplification.

Briefly, 0.12 - 0.40 μg of RNA was incubated with gene specific oligonucleotides (0.2 μM final primer concentration) in a 25 μL volume containing 12.5 μL of 2x Reaction Mix (1.6 mM $MgSO_4$ and 200 μM dNTP) and 1 U SuperScript™ III RT/ Platinum® *Taq* Mix (Invitrogen) for 30min at 56-60 °C. After reverse transcription the samples were initially denatured for 2 min at 94 °C. The reactions were then amplified for 25 - 40 PCR cycles that included a 94 °C denaturation step for 15 s, 55 - 60 °C annealing step for 30 s, and a 68 °C extension step for 60 s, with a final extension time of 5 min at 68 °C. As an internal control, the house keeping genes *β-actin* or *GAPDH* were amplified from the same samples. All RT-PCR products were separated *via* electrophoresis on a 1% agarose gel in 1x TAE buffer and visualised with EtBr staining.

2.5 DETECTION OF PROTEIN USING WESTERN BLOT ANALYSIS

2.5.1 Extraction of Protein from Animal Tissues

Tissues removed from euthanased mice were rinsed in PBS to remove excess blood, snap frozen in liquid nitrogen and stored at -80 °C. When required for analysis, tissue samples were thawed on ice and 500 μL of freshly prepared, ice-cold lysis solution [150 mM NaCl, 10 mM tris-HCl (pH 7.4), 1.5 % triton X-100, 0.5% SDS, 1 mM EDTA, 1mM EGTA, 0.04mM NaF and complete protease inhibitor®] added. Tissues samples were homogenised in lysis solution using sterile tissue grinders and incubated on ice for 30 min. The samples were then subjected to multiple 2 sec bursts of sonication on ice and centrifuged at 14 000 rpm for 45 min at 4 °C. The protein lysate supernatants were retained and protein concentrations determined using the bicinchoninic acid protein assay reagent (Progen Biosciences, Brisbane, Australia) according to the manufacturer's directions.

2.5.2 Western Blot Analysis

Protein lysates were first heat denatured at 90 °C for 1 min. To separate proteins, sodium dodecyl sulphate-polyacrylamide gel electrophoresis (SDS-PAGE) was carried out using the NuPAGE® system as per the manufacturer's instructions (Invitrogen). Briefly, samples were loaded (50 – 100 μg/lane) alongside protein size standards (BioRad, Sydney, Australia) onto a 4-12% NuPAGE® Bis-Tris gel (Invitrogen). Electrophoresis was carried out at 200 V for 45 – 60 min in 1x MES SDS running buffer (Invitrogen). Proteins were then electroblotted at 30 V for 2 h onto a polyvinyl difluoride membrane in NuPAGE® transfer buffer (Invitrogen). Membranes were then blocked overnight in 5% skim milk powder in 1x TBS buffer containing 0.1% tween (Sigma-Aldrich) (TBS-T) on a platform rocker (Edwards Instruments, Thebarton, Australia).

The next day, membranes were incubated with primary antibodies in 5% skim milk powder and 1x TBS-T for 2 h at room temperature. This step, and all further antibody incubation and washing steps were performed on a platform rocker (Edwards Instruments). Following primary antibody incubation, membranes were washed four times for 5 min each with 1x TBS-T and incubated with secondary antibodies for 1 h at room temperature. Membranes were then washed three times with 1x TBS-T and one time with 1x TBS for 5 min each. After washing, membranes were developed using the Enhanced Chemiluminescence Plus™ western blot detection reagent (Amersham Biosciences, Buckinghamshire, UK) and exposed to X-ray film (Kodak, New York, USA). Film was developed using a Konica-Minolta SRX-101A film processor (Konica-Minolta, Sydney, Australia). As an internal control for protein loading, membranes were also probed for GAPDH (Santa Cruz Biotechnology, Santa Cruz, USA).

2.6 IRP-RNA BINDING ACTIVITY

2.6.1 Extraction of Protein from Animal Tissue

Tissue extracts were prepared using established protocols (Nie et al., 2005). Briefly, heart tissue harvested from euthanased mice was rinsed in PBS to remove excess blood. Tissue lysates were prepared at 4 °C in 80 µL of freshly prepared Munro buffer   (3mM $MgCl_2$, 40 mM KCl, 5% glycerol, 10 mM HEPES, 1 mM dithiothreitol, pH 7.6) with 0.2% Nonidet-P40 (NP40; Roche) using vigorous pipetting. Lysates were then gently mixed at 4 °C in 160 µL of freshly prepared Munro buffer (in the absence of NP40), centrifuged at 10,000 rpm for 3 min at 4 °C, and the cytoplasmic protein extract (supernatant) collected.

2.6.2 Gel Retardation Analysis

Gel retardation assays were performed by Dr. Marc Mikhael (Lady Davis Institute, McGill University, Montreal, Canada) using standard techniques (Nie et al., 2005). In these assays, protein extracts (Section 2.6.1) were incubated with ^{32}P-labelled IRE-RNA probes to initiate IRP-IRE binding interactions. The resultant RNA-protein complexes were analysed using nondenaturing PAGE gels. To maximally activate IRP-RNA binding activity, simultaneous experiments were performed using 2% β-mercaptoethanol (β-ME; Sigma-Aldrich) to treat protein extracts prior to incubation with ^{32}P-RNA probe.

2.7 IN VIVO *ADMINISTRATION OF* ^{59}*FE AND CELLULAR FRACTIONATION*

To examine the intracellular distribution of iron *in vivo*, mice were intravenously (i.v.) injected with 0.6 mg of ^{59}Fe-Tf (prepared as in Section 2.1.3) *via* the tail vein. Between 2-96 h post i.v. injection, hearts were removed and washed in ice-cold sucrose-tris buffer (ST; 250 mM sucrose, 10 mM tris-HCl, pH 7.4 supplemented with complete protease inhibitor$^{®}$) to remove excess blood. Hearts were homogenised in ice-cold ST buffer using a Dounce tissue grinder (Sigma-Aldrich) and centrifuged at 800 g/10 min/4 °C to isolate the cytosolic and mitochondrial fractions (supernatant) from the nuclear fraction and debris (pellet). The supernatant was collected and further centrifuged at 16,000 g/45 min/4 °C to separate the cytosol (supernatant) from the stromal mitochondrial membrane (pellet).

2.8 ANALYSIS OF RESULTS AND DATA

2.8.1 Densitometry

Densitometric analysis was performed to quantify the intensities of bands produced from RT-PCR, western blotting and IRP-RNA binding activity assays. Films were scanned and consequently analysed using the densitometric software, Quantity One (BioRad). For RT-PCR and western blotting, the relative intensity of protein bands were expressed as a proportion of β-actin or GAPDH loading controls.

2.8.2 Statistics

Data is expressed as mean ± standard deviation (SD) or as mean ± standard error of the mean (SEM) as indicated for each experiment. Experimental data were compared using Student's t-test. Results were considered statistically significant when $p < 0.05$.

CHAPTER 3

A CLASS OF IRON CHELATORS WITH A WIDE SPECTRUM OF POTENT ANTI-TUMOUR ACTIVITY THAT OVERCOME RESISTANCE TO CHEMOTHERAPEUTICS

THIS CHAPTER CONTAINS WORK PUBLISHED IN:

Whitnall M, Howard J, Ponka P and Richardson DR (2006) A class of iron chelators with a wide spectrum of potent antitumour activity that overcomes resistance to chemotherapeutics. *Proc Natl Acad Sci USA* 103(40):14901-06.

3.1 INTRODUCTION

Depriving cancer cells of the essential nutrient iron is a novel approach for the treatment of cancer (Buss et al., 2004, Kalinowski and Richardson, 2005, Le and Richardson, 2002). Iron-containing proteins perform key reactions involved in energy metabolism and DNA synthesis. Indeed, the rate-limiting step of DNA synthesis is catalysed by the iron-containing enzyme, ribonucleotide reductase (Thelander and Reichard, 1979). Moreover, chelators such as desferrioxamine (DFO; Figure 3.1A) arrest cells at the G_1/S interface, inhibiting cell-cycle progression and inducing apoptosis (Brodie et al., 1993, Richardson and Milnes, 1997).

Many *in vitro* and *in vivo* studies have shown that compared to normal cells, cancer cells are more sensitive to iron deprivation because of their marked iron requirements (Buss et al., 2004, Kalinowski and Richardson, 2005, Le and Richardson, 2002). To facilitate rapid replication, neoplastic cells have significantly higher levels of ribonucleotide reductase and TfR1 (Buss et al., 2004, Kalinowski and Richardson, 2005). The higher iron utilisation by cancer cells than their normal counterparts provides a rationale for the selective anti-tumour activity of chelators (Buss et al., 2004, Kalinowski and Richardson, 2005, Le and Richardson, 2002).

To date, the only chelator in widespread use for the treatment of iron overload disease is DFO. In addition, DFO also has some anti-tumour activity (Buss et al., 2004, Kalinowski and Richardson, 2005, Le and Richardson, 2002). Recently, the iron chelator, Triapine (3-aminopyridine-2-carboxaldehyde thiosemicarbazone; Figure 3.1A), which inhibits ribonucleotide reductase activity and tumour growth *in vitro* and *in vivo* (Finch et al., 2000), has entered phase I and II clinical trials (Buss et al.,

2004, Kalinowski and Richardson, 2005). Additionally, some chelators of the pyridoxal isonicotinoyl hydrazone (PIH) class (Ponka et al., 1979a) possess potent anti-tumour activity *e.g.*, 2-hydroxy-1-naphthylaldehyde isonicotinoyl hydrazone (311) (Richardson et al., 1995).

Studies of the structure-activity relationships of the PIH analogues led to the development of several novel series of chelators showing significantly greater activity, the most effective being the di-2-pyridylketone thiosemicarbazone (DpT; Figure 3.1B) and di-2-pyridylketone isonicotinoyl hydrazone (PKIH; Figure 3.1C) analogues (Becker et al., 2003, Yuan et al., 2004). From preliminary screening, one of the most efficient of these chelators identified was di-2-pyridylketone-4,4,-dimethyl-3-thiosemicarbazone (Dp44mT; Figure 3.1B). This ligand showed selective anti-tumour activity and inhibited murine M109 lung carcinoma growth *in vivo* by 47% in 5 days (Yuan et al., 2004). The cytotoxic mechanism of action of this chelator involved not only iron chelation, but also redox cycling of its iron complex to generate ROS (Yuan et al., 2004). Moreover, in cultured cells, Dp44mT resulted in marked up-regulation of the iron-responsive tumour growth and metastasis suppressor, *NDRG1* (*N-myc downstream regulated gene-1*) (Le and Richardson, 2004). Up-regulation of *NDRG1* suppresses primary tumour growth and metastasis (Bandyopadhyay et al., 2003, Kurdistani et al., 1998), and may be another mechanism by which chelators inhibit cancer cell proliferation.

Herein the *in vitro*, and in particular, *in vivo* anti-tumour activity of our most effective DpT and PKIH chelators against human tumours, was investigated. Notably, these studies demonstrate the broad-spectrum activity of these chelators against a wide range of cancer cell types *in vitro* and *in vivo*, including those possessing multi-drug resistant phenotypes.

57

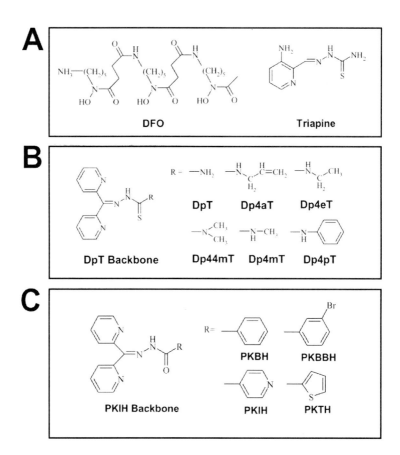

Figure 3.1 Chemical structures of key iron chelators used in this study.
(A) Desferrioxamine (DFO) and Triapine, **(B)** the di-2-pyridylketone
thiosemicarbazone (DpT) backbone and DpT analogues, and **(C)** the di-2-
pyridylketone isonicotinoyl hydrazone (PKIH) backbone and PKIH
analogues.

3.2 MATERIALS AND METHODS

3.2.1 Chelators and Cytotoxics

DFO was purchased from Novartis (Basel, Switzerland). Triapine was a gift from Vion Pharmaceuticals (New Haven, USA). The DpT and PKIH analogues were synthesised using standard procedures (Richardson et al., 2006).

Doxorubicin (DOX) was purchased from Pharmacia (Sydney, Australia). Etoposide and vincristine were purchased from Sigma-Aldrich.

3.2.2 Cell culture

The human cell lines SK-N-MC neuroepithelioma, IMR-32 neuroblastoma, NCI H2452, NCI H2052 and MSTO 211H mesothelioma, DU 145, LNCaP, PC-3, 22Rv1 and LNCaP CHUNG prostate cancer, Hep G2 hepatoma, H69AR, DMS-53 and NCI H2126 lung carcinoma, HeLa cervical cancer, T47D breast cancer, K562 and CCRF-CEM leukemic cells and SK-Mel-28 melanoma, were obtained from the American Type Culture Collection (Manassas, USA). The human Kelly neuroblastoma cell line was obtained from the European Collection of Cell Cultures (Wiltshire, UK). The human HUH7 hepatoma and CFPAC-1 pancreatic cancer lines were provided by Dr. Mohammad Pourgholami (St. George Hospital, Sydney, Australia). The human A2780 ovarian carcinoma cell line was a gift from Prof. Susan Clark (Garvan Institute, Sydney, Australia). The following human cancer cell lines were donated by Dr. Richard Lock (Children's Cancer Institute Australia, Sydney, Australia): MCF-7 breast cancer cells and their etoposide-resistant subclone MCF-7/VP (maintained in 4 μM etoposide); KB3-1 epidermoid carcinoma cells and their vinblastine-resistant subclone KB-V1 (maintained in 0.1 μM vinblastine); and ALL3, ALL7 and ALL19 leukemic cells.

The SK-Mel-28 cell line was grown in Eagle's minimum essential media (MEM; Gibco, Sydney, Australia). The HUH7, CFPAC-1, MCF-7, MCF-7/VP, KB3-1 and KB-V1 cell lines were grown in Dulbecco's modified Eagle medium (DMEM; Gibco). All remaining cell lines were grown in RPMI-1640 media (Gibco). The following supplements were added to all culture media: 10% (v/v) foetal bovine serum (Gibco), 1% (v/v) non-essential amino acids (Gibco), 1% (v/v) sodium pyruvate (Gibco), 2 mM L-glutamine (Gibco), 100 μg/mL streptomycin (Gibco), 100 U/mL penicillin (Gibco), and 0.28 μg/mL fungizone (Squibb Pharmaceuticals, Montr, Canada).

Cells were grown in an incubator (Forma Scientific, Ohio, USA) at 37 °C in a humidified atmosphere of 5% CO_2/95% air and sub-cultured as described previously (Richardson and Baker, 1990). Cellular growth and viability were assessed by phase contrast microscopy, cell adherence to the culture substratum, and Trypan blue staining (Sigma-Aldrich).

3.2.3 MTT Cell Proliferation Assay

Cellular proliferation was examined using the MTT (3-4,5-dimethylthiazol-2,5 diphenyl tetrabromide) assay following a similar method as described previously (Richardson et al., 1995). In this method, MTT is reduced in viable cells by mitochondrial dehydrogenase to a purple coloured crystal, formazan, allowing cell viability to be determined by a colourimetric assay. Cells were seeded in 96-well microtitre plates in 0.1 mL of appropriate media (as per Section 3.2.2). Seeding densities, determined from cellular growth rate as observed in culture, were: 5,000 cells/well for IMR-32, NCI H2452 and PC-3 cell lines; 10,000 cells/well for Kelly, NCI H2052, MSTO 211H, DU 145, HepG2, HeLa, T47D, MCF7, MCF-7/VP, CCRF-CEM and SK-Mel-28 cell lines and; 15,000 cells/well for SK-N-MC, LNCaP, 22Rv1, LNCaP CHUNG, HUH7, H69AR, DMS-53, NCI H2126, CFPAC-1, KB3-1, KB-V1, A2780, ALL 3, ALL 7 and ALL 19 cell lines. These seeding densities resulted in exponential growth of the cells for the duration of the assay. After seeding, cells were incubated overnight at 37 °C.

Following overnight attachment, DpT and PKIH analogues were dissolved in dimethyl sulfoxide (DMSO; Sigma-Aldrich) and added to the cells in 0.1 mL of media containing 1.25 μM ^{56}Fe-Tf (prepared as described in Section 2.1.3). The iron chelators 311 (dissolved in DMSO), DFO (dissolved in media) and Triapine (dissolved in DMSO) were included as internal positive controls along with the clinically used cytotoxic agent, DOX (prepared in media). Cells were then incubated for a further 48 h at 37 °C.

After incubation, 10 μL of MTT was added to the cells (5 mg/mL made up in PBS) which were then incubated for a final period of 2 h at 37 °C. After this, the media was carefully aspirated from the wells and replaced with 100 μL of MTT lysis buffer (50% isobutanol, 40 mM HCl, 10% SDS) to lyse cells and release formazan. The absorbance of each well was then read at 570 nm using a Victor^3™ V Multilabel Counter plate reader (PerkinElmer).

3.2.4 Colony Formation Assay

Standard procedures were used to perform clonogenic assays (Abeysinghe et al., 2001) using A2780 ovarian carcinoma and SK-N-MC neuroepithelioma cells. Cells were seeded into 24-well plates at a density of 100 cells/well to allow for exponential growth. After overnight attachment and incubation at 37 °C, cells were treated with Dp44mT or the reference controls DFO or DOX (prepared as in Section 3.2.3) and incubated for a further 72 h. Following this, the chelator/DOX-containing medium was aspirated from the cells and replaced with fresh media. Colonies were allowed to form for 10-15 days, after which cells were fixed for 3 min with 3.7% paraformaldehyde in PBS and stained for 10 min with 0.1% crystal violet (Sigma-Aldrich). Colonies with > 50 cells were counted manually under a microscope.

3.2.5 Tumour Xenografts in Nude Mice and Chelator Administration

Female BALB/c nu/nu mice (Animal Resources Centre, Canning Vale, Australia) were used at 8-10 weeks of age. Tumour cells in culture were harvested and 1×10^7 cells were suspended in Matrigel (BD Biosciences) and injected subcutaneously into the right flanks of mice. After engraftment, tumour size was monitored and measurements made using Vernier callipers. Tumour volumes were calculated using the following standard formula, where (d) is the shortest width and (D) is the longest length: tumour volume $(mm^3) = (d)^2 \times (D)/2$ (Balsari et al., 2004). When tumour volumes reached 120 mm^3, i.v. treatment began (day 0) using the chelators, Dp44mT and Triapine dissolved in 15% propylene glycol in 0.9% saline. I.v. chelator injections were administered over 5 consecutive days per week for up to 7 weeks. Control mice were treated with vehicle alone.

After 2-7 weeks of treatment, mice were sacrificed, tissues and blood harvested and organ weights assessed (Section 2.2.2). Blood was used for haematological analysis (as per Section 2.3.1) and analysis of serum chemistry and blood cell morphology (as below). Harvested tissues were used for histochemistry (as per Section 2.3.3), measurement of tissue iron stores (as per Section 2.3.2) and RT-PCR analysis (as below).

3.2.6 Serum Biochemistry and Blood Cell Morphology

Blood taken from anaesthetised mice *via* cardiac puncture, was added to serum chemistry tubes containing a clot activator (BD Biosciences). Tubes were centrifuged for 15 min at 7500 rpm to separate out the serum. Serum biochemistry parameters were determined using a Konelab 20i analyser (Thermo Electron Corporation, Vantaa, Finland).

Additionally, blood smears were also prepared, and May-Grünwald/Giemsa stains kindly performed by Ms Elaine Chew (Faculty of Veterinary Science, University of Sydney, Sydney, Australia) for microscopic analysis.

3.2.7 Gene Expression Analysis

To assess *NDRG1*, *TfR1* and *VEGF1* mRNA expression, RNA was isolated from liver and tumour tissue as described in Section 2.4.1, and semiquantitative RT-PCR performed as per Section 2.4.2 using the specific primers listed in Table 3.1. The house-keeping gene, *β-actin*, was used as an RNA loading control. Densitometric analysis was performed as per Section 2.8.1

Table 3.1 Sequences and accession numbers of primers used to amplify RNA extracted from human tumour xenografts and mouse liver tissue.

Primer Name	Accession No.	Oligonucleotides (5' – 3')		Product size (bp)
		Forward	Reverse	
hNDRG1	NM_006096	CCCTCGCGTTA GGCAGGTGA	AGGGGTACATG TACCCTGCG	370
hTfR1	X01060	TCAGGTCAAAG ACAGCGCTCAA AACTC	AGTCTCCTTCCA TATTCCCAAAC AGCTTTT	488
hVEGF1	NM_00102536 6	CCATGCCAAGT GGTCC	AAATGCTTTCTC CGCTCT	525
hβ-actin	NM_001101	CCCGCCGCCAG CTCACCATGG	AAGGTCTCAAA CATGATCTGGG TC	397
mNDRG1	NM_010884	TGCTTGCTCATT AGGTGTGTGAT AGC	CCATCCTGAGA TCTTAGAGGCA GC	581
mTfR1	NM_011638	TCCCGAGGGTT ATGTGGC	GGCGGAAACTG AGTATGATTGA	307
mVEGF1	NM_009505	CCATGCCAAGT GGTCC	AAATGCTTTCTC CGCTCT	399
mβ-actin	NM_007393	CCCGCCACCAG TTCGCCATGG	AAGGTCTCAAA CATGATCTGGG TC	397

3.3 RESULTS

3.3.1 DpT and PKIH Iron Chelators Show High Anti-proliferative Activity Against a Range of Tumour Cell Lines

Previously, the high anti-proliferative activity of chelators of the DpT and PKIH classes of ligands were shown in a limited number of cell lines (Becker et al., 2003, Yuan et al., 2004). Herein, 28 cell types were examined to determine the spectrum of anti-tumour activity of the most effective DpT and PKIH analogues (Table 3.2). DFO, 311 and Triapine, and the cytotoxic agent DOX were included as positive controls.

Of the 12 chelators tested, the least effective was DFO, with an IC_{50} value that ranged from 3 to >25 μM (Table 3.2). Dp44mT showed the greatest anti-tumour efficacy with an IC_{50} that ranged from 0.005 - 0.4 μM. The average IC_{50} of Dp44mT over the 28 cell types was 0.03 $\pm$ 0.01 μM, which was significantly lower than that of the clinically-trialled chelator, Triapine (average IC_{50}: 1.41 $\pm$ 0.37 μM). Moreover, the anti-proliferative activity of Dp44mT was greater than the established cytotoxic agent, DOX, in 26 of 28 cell lines. In fact, the average IC_{50} of DOX in the 28 cell types was 0.62 $\pm$ 0.35 μM. Related compounds to Dp44mT, namely PKBBH (di-2-pyridylketone 3-bromobenzoyl hydrazone), PKIH, PKTH (di-2-pyridlketone thiophenecarboxyl hydrazone), Dp4aT (di-2-pyridlketone 4-allyl-3-thiosemicarbazone), Dp4eT (di-2-pyridlketone 4-ethyl-3-thiosemicarbazone), Dp4mT (di-2-pyridlketone 4-methyl-3-thiosemicarbazone) and Dp4pT (di-2-pyridlketone 4-phenyl-3-thiosemicarbazone) (average IC_{50} over 25 - 28 cell lines = 0.57, 1.03, 0.88, 0.61, 0.77, 1.70 and 0.20 μM, respectively) also demonstrated appreciable activity that was not significantly different from DOX. The anti-proliferative activity of Dp44mT was significantly more effective than all of the latter compounds.

Table 3.2 IC$_{50}$ values of DpT and PKIH chelators as compared to DFO, DOX, Triapine and 311 in various human tumour cell lines

CELL LINE	TUMOUR TYPE	p53 status	IC$_{50}$ (μM) VALUES												
			DFO	DOX	Triapine	311	PKIH	PKTH	PKBH	PKBBH	Dp4aT	Dp4eT	Dp4mT	Dp4pT	Dp44mT
SK-N-MC	Neuro-epithelioma	mu[1]	10.52	0.02	0.30	1.38	0.65	0.65	3.13	0.30	0.04	0.09	2.77	0.02	0.01
IMR-32	Neuro-blastoma	wt[2]	5.47	0.01	0.13	0.30	0.34	0.18	0.76	0.03	0.01	0.03	0.01	0.01	0.02
Kelly		wt[3]	3.30	0.02	0.36	0.75	0.47	0.64	1.17	0.29	0.01	0.03	0.08	0.01	0.01
NCI H2452	Meso-thelioma	?	>25	0.17	0.82	0.47	0.86	0.73	1.29	0.21	0.03	1.17	1.86	0.01	0.009
NCI H2052		?	21.88	0.02	0.68	0.73	1.17	1.17	2.13	0.32	0.02	0.04	0.35	0.006	0.006
MSTO 211H		wt[4]	8.08	0.06	0.43	0.92	1.15	0.64	>6.25	0.46	2.34	0.42	>6.25	0.06	0.02
DU 145		mu[5]	12.58	0.06	0.61	1.68	0.56	1.21	2.66	0.18	2.50	4.40	6.99	1.53	0.05
LNCaP	Prostate	wt[6]	12.62	0.13	1.13	0.88	0.32	0.72	2.19	0.24	0.04	0.10	1.10	0.01	0.008
PC-3		mu[7]	3.94	0.10	0.51	0.39	0.43	0.37	2.35	0.17	0.17	0.06	0.66	0.03	0.007
22Rv1		wt[6]	9.34	0.08	0.78	1.19	1.19	1.17	4.40	0.30	0.04	0.07	0.79	0.02	0.01
LNCaP CHUNG		?	>25	0.08	1.29	1.21	>6.25	0.7	0.78	1.21	1.09	0.53	6.25	0.03	0.008
Hep G2	Hepatoma	wt[8]	4.60	0.80	1.23	0.62	0.56	0.44	4.92	0.3	0.01	0.01	0.07	0.007	0.007
HUH7		mu[8]	3.11	0.16	-	0.54	0.88	0.55	3.32	0.26	0.4	0.05	0.26	0.17	0.01
H69AR	Lung	?	14.5	3.91	5.47	2.00	1.46	0.61	>6.25	0.59	5.47	4.92	>6.25	1.21	0.04
DMS-53		?	9.38	0.22	1.19	0.72	0.74	0.78	>6.25	0.63	0.02	0.07	0.05	0.03	0.009
NCI H2126		mu[9]	>25	0.92	5.63	1.23	1.82	1.68	3.64	5.16	0.46	0.72	5.08	0.06	0.09
CFPAC-1	Pancreas	mu[10]	15.75	0.21	0.77	1.37	1.37	1.07	0.35	0.27	2.75	3.91	>6.25	0.79	0.40
HeLa	Cervical	wt[11]	>25	0.01	1.11	1.30	0.78	1.30	>6.25	0.52	0.13	0.08	1.46	0.02	0.008
T47D	Breast	mu[12]	18.44	0.04	0.78	0.68	1.98	1.14	1.95	0.18	0.01	0.02	0.01	0.009	0.009
MCF-7		wt[12]	12.50	0.24	1.17	0.78	1.56	0.78	2.40	0.39	0.05	0.04	0.20	0.01	0.01
KB3-1	Naso-pharyngeal	?	20.80	8.96	>6.25	1.81	2.15	2.05	19.38	0.54	0.93	2.96	5.00	0.30	0.05
A2780	Ovarian	wt[12]	9.20	0.01	0.60	0.83	0.59	0.54	4.10	0.30	0.01	0.005	0.06	0.05	0.005
K562		mu[13]	>25	0.10	1.07	2.35	1.46	0.98	5.47	0.39	0.29	0.73	0.69	0.05	0.01
CCRF-CEM	Leukemia	mu[12]	5.63	0.03	0.47	0.39	0.78	0.51	3.82	0.16	0.01	0.01	0.07	0.006	0.006
ALL 3		wt[14]	>25	0.03	4.38	0.79	-	-	-	-	0.07	0.08	-	0.02	0.006
ALL 7		wt[14]	23.13	0.14	1.56	1.27	-	-	-	-	0.05	0.08	-	0.02	0.007
ALL 19		wt[14]	15.00	0.08	2.42	1.26	-	-	-	-	0.02	0.06	-	0.007	0.007
SK-Mel-28	Melanoma	wt[15]	10.77	0.77	1.88	0.79	1.56	1.41	3.60	0.89	0.02	0.97	3.49	1.22	0.009

Abbreviations: mu, mutant p53; wt, wild-type p53; ? denotes unknown p53 status.

Results are expressed as the mean of 2 independent experiments with duplicates in each experiment.

Superscripted numbers denote cited reference for p53 status as below:

1. (Liang and Richardson, 2003)
2. (Gangopadhyay et al., 2002)
3. (Woessmann et al., 2002)
4. (Yang et al., 2001)
5. (Ioffe et al., 2004)
6. (Cronauer et al., 2004)
7. (O'Connor et al., 1997)
8. (Chi et al., 2004)
9. (Carretero et al., 2004)
10. (Kokkinakis et al., 2003)
11. (Toyozumi et al., 2004)
12. (Lu et al., 2001)
13. (Usuda et al., 2003)
14. (Lock et al., 2002)
15. (Dong et al., 1999)

3.3.2 Clonogenic Assays with Dp44mT

Clonogenic assays were used to assess the anti-tumour efficacy of Dp44mT. Figure 3.2A shows the response of A2780 cells to a 48 h exposure to DFO, DOX or Dp44mT. Even at the highest concentration of DFO (20 μM) or DOX (0.02 μM), colonies survived. In contrast, at its lowest concentration, Dp44mT (0.00125 μM) inhibited survival of A2780 clones by approximately 50% compared with the control. At 0.0025 μM, Dp44mT completely prevented colony formation (Figure 3.2A). Similar results were obtained for SK-N-MC cells (data not shown).

3.3.3 Dp44mT Retains Anti-proliferative Activity in Drug-Resistant Cell Lines

Resistance of tumour cells to established chemotherapeutic agents is a marked clinical problem (Aouali et al., 2005). Hence, Dp44mT was assessed for its ability to overcome multi-drug resistant mechanisms in etoposide-resistant MCF-7/VP (Schneider et al., 1994) clones of MCF-7 breast cancer cells and vinblastine-resistant KB-V1 (Akiyama et al., 1985, Shen et al., 1986) clones of KB3-1 epidermoid carcinoma cells. To confirm resistance was maintained, etoposide (Figure 3.2B) and vinblastine (Figure 3.2C) were included as relevant controls. Etoposide-sensitive and -resistant cells were equally susceptible to the effects of Dp44mT, both resulting in an IC_{50} of 0.012 μM (Figure 3.2B). These results indicate that resistance to etoposide did not interfere with the efficacy of Dp44mT.

Interestingly, vinblastine-resistant KB-V1 cells were more susceptible to Dp44mT than the vinblastine-sensitive parental cell line, KB3-1 (Figure

3.2C). As expected, the KB-V1 cell type remained resistant to vinblastine compared with the sensitive parental cells (KB3-1; Figure 3.2C). These results show that Dp44mT can overcome resistance to vinblastine.

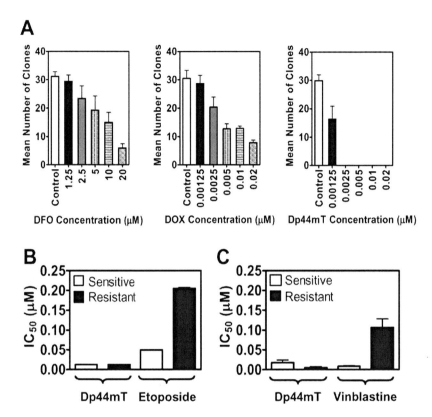

Figure 3.2   Dp44mT markedly inhibits clonogenic formation and overcomes resistance to other cytotoxic agents. (A) Dp44mT is more effective than   DFO and DOX at preventing clonogenic formation in A2780 human ovarian carcinoma. Cells were   treated with chelators or DOX for 48 h, and outgrowth was assessed after 10-15 days in agent-free medium. **(B)** The MCF-7/VP cell line is resistant to etoposide compared with their sensitive parental counterpart, MCF-7. In contrast, the anti-proliferative activity of Dp44mT was equally potent in these cells. **(C)** KB-V1 cells are resistant to vinblastine compared with their parental counterpart, KB3-1, whereas the anti-proliferative activity of Dp44mT is greater in the resistant clone than the sensitive cell. Results are mean ± SD from three experiments.

3.3.4 Sensitivity of Tumour Cells to DpT Chelators is Independent of p53 Status

Because numerous tumours contain functionally defective p53, anti-cancer agents that induce apoptosis in a p53-independent manner must be developed (Abeysinghe et al., 2001, Guimaraes and Hainaut, 2002, Lowe, 1995, O'Connor et al., 1997). Hence, the ability of the DpT chelators to act independent of p53 apoptotic pathways was examined. For all chelators, there was no correlation between p53 status and $-logIC_{50}$ (data not shown), indicating that chelators act via a p53-independent mechanism to inhibit proliferation.

3.3.5 Dp44mT Markedly Inhibits the Growth of Human Tumour Xenografts *In Vivo*

3.3.5.1 Short-Term Studies

Figures 3.3A-C show the effects of short-term Dp44mT treatment on the growth of established xenografts in mice. Much higher doses of Triapine (a positive control) than Dp44mT were required to observe significant anti-tumour activity. After 2 weeks of treatment, the average net tumour size of DMS-53 xenografts in control mice was 267 mm^3, whereas in Dp44mT (0.75 mg/kg/day)-treated mice, it was significantly reduced to 15 mm^3 (Figure 3.3A). Notably, Dp44mT at a 16-fold lower dose (0.75 mg/kg/day), showed significantly greater anti-tumour activity than Triapine (12 mg/kg/day). A similar response to Dp44mT was also observed in SK-N-MC and SK-Mel-28 xenografts (Figures 3.3B and C, respectively).

3.3.5.2 Long-Term Studies

Rapid growth of SK-N-MC and DMS-53 xenografts meant that for ethical reasons they could not be used for long-term studies, because the tumours in control mice became ulcerated after 2 weeks. In contrast, SK-Mel-28 xenografts grew at a slower rate, allowing an extended treatment for 7 weeks (Figure 3.3D).

Average net tumour size in Dp44mT (0.4 mg/kg/)-treated mice (49 mm^3) was significantly smaller than in control mice (612 mm^3) after 7 weeks (Figures 3.3D and E). Tumour regression was also observed in mice treated with 0.75 mg/kg/day of Dp44mT. However, after 3 weeks of treatment at this latter dose, mice experienced a 14% decrease in body weight, and for ethical reasons, were culled. In contrast, at 0.4 mg/kg/day, Dp44mT was well tolerated, with weight loss in mice not exceeding 10% over 7 weeks (see Section 3.3.6, below).

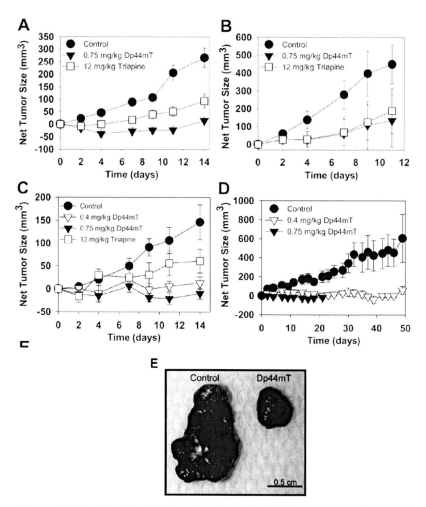

Figure 3.3 Dp44mT is highly effective at inhibiting growth of a range of human xenografts in nude mice. Dp44mT (0.75 mg/kg/day) is equally or more effective than Triapine at inhibiting growth of **(A)** DMS-53 lung carcinoma, **(B)** SK-N-MC neuroepithelioma, and **(C)** SK-Mel-28 melanoma xenografts when administered i.v. once per day, 5 days/week for up to 2 weeks. Each point represents mean ± SEM from 6-12 mice. **(D)** Dp44mT (0.4 or 0.7 mg/kg/day) inhibits SK-Mel-28 melanoma xenografts when given i.v. once per day for up to 7 weeks. Each point represents mean ± SEM from 6 mice. **(E)** Photograph of SK-Mel-28 melanoma tumours taken from mice after 7 weeks of treatment with the vehicle control or Dp44mT (0.4 mg/kg/day) using the regimen in (D).

3.3.6 Biological Assessment Following Chelator Treatment

Because Dp44mT is an iron chelator (Yuan et al., 2004), the effects Dp44mT may have on physiological processes was assessed. After 2 weeks, Dp44mT (0.75 mg/kg/day)-treated mice experienced significant ($p < 0.001$) weight loss compared to control animals (Table 3.3). However, no significant difference in weight loss was observed between mice receiving the lower dose of Dp44mT (0.4 mg/kg/day) and the controls after 7 weeks of treatment (Table 3.4).

There was a significant ($p < 0.01$) increase in platelets and a slight but not significant increase in red blood cell (RBC) counts in mice treated for 2 weeks with Dp44mT (0.75 mg/kg/day) compared with controls (Table 3.3). A significant ($p < 0.05$) decrease in RBC counts was observed in mice treated with Triapine (Table 3.3). Importantly, no significant differences in haematological indices were found in mice using the lower Dp44mT dose (0.4 mg/kg/day; Table 3.4) over 7 weeks.

After short-term treatment with Dp44mT (0.75 mg/kg/day) or vehicle control, no significant differences were detected in a range of serum biochemical parameters including creatine kinase in muscle and brain, aspartate aminotransferase, lactate dehydrogenase, alkaline phosphatase, alanine aminotransferase, total bilirubin, total protein, creatinine and glucose (data not shown). However, mice treated with Triapine experienced a marked increase in alkaline phosphatase (185 ± 8, $n = 3$) compared to the control (115 ± 10, $n = 3$).

Table 3.3 Weight loss and haematological indices of mice treated with vehicle control, Dp44mT or Triapine in animals bearing human DMS-53 lung carcinoma xenografts treated for 2 weeks.

	Experimental Groups[a]		
	Control	*Dp44mT* *(0.75 mg/kg/day)*	*Triapine* *(12 mg/kg/day)*
Body weight loss (% of total weight)	2.1 ± 0.8 (27)	8.3 ± 1.04 (24)[b]	2.9 ± 1.1 (27)
RBC (x 10^{12}/L)	8.9 ± 0.3 (14)	9.2 ± 0.2 (13)	7.7 ± 0.4 (11)[c]
Hb (g/L)	14.9 ± 0.3 (14)	14.8 ± 0.3 (13)	13.3 ± 0.7 (11)
Hct	0.44 ± 0.01 (14)	0.45 ± 0.01 (13)	0.40 ± 0.02 (11)
Platelets (x 10^9/L)	636.8 ± 136 (8)	1153.4 ± 138.1(11)[d]	530.8 ± 65.2 (9)
WBC (x 10^9/L)	4.4 ± 0.6 (14)	4.8 ± 0.4 (13)	6.2 ± 1.6 (9)

[a] Data are expressed as mean ± SEM for (*n*) mice
[b] $p < 0.001$ compared with control.
[c] $p < 0.05$ compared with control.
[d] $p < 0.01$ compared with control

Abbreviations: RBC, red blood cell; Hb, haemoglobin; Hct, haematocrit; WBC, white blood cell.

Table 3.4 Weight loss and haematological indices of mice treated with vehicle control or Dp44mT in animals bearing human SK-Mel-28 melanoma xenografts treated for 7 weeks.

	Experimental Groups[a]	
	Control	*Dp44mT* *(0.4 mg/kg/day)*
Body weight loss (% of total weight)	2.9 ± 1.5 (5)	3.3 ± 1.5 (4)
RBC (x 10^{12}/L)	9.5 ± 0.1 (5)	9.7 ± 0.3 (4)
Hb (g/L)	14.7 ± 0.2 (5)	14.2 ± 0.1 (4)
Hct	0.40 ± 0.01 (5)	0.43 ± 0.01 (4)
Platelets (x 10^{9}/L)	859.6 ± 146.6 (5)	782.3 ± 168.4 (4)
WBC (x 10^{9}/L)	7.7 ± 2.9 (5)	10.2 ± 1.6 (4)

[a] Data are expressed as mean ± SEM for (*n*) mice.

Abbreviations: RBC, red blood cell; Hb, haemoglobin; Hct, haematocrit; WBC, white blood cell.

3.3.7 Organ Weights and Tissue Iron Levels After Chelator Treatment

No significant changes were found in organ-to-total-body-weight ratios in tumour-bearing mice comparing Dp44mT and control mice after short-term treatment (data not shown). In contrast, Triapine caused a significant increase (1.7-fold) in splenic weight when expressed as a percentage of total body weight (1.02 ± 0.06 %, $n = 25$) compared to control mice ($0.6 \pm 0.03\%$, $n = 27$). In the long-term group, a significant increase in heart weight was observed after Dp44mT (0.4 mg/kg/day) ($0.8 \pm 0.06\%$, $n = 4$) compared to control mice ($0.5 \pm 0.01\%$, $n = 6$).

In short-term studies, there was a significant ($p < 0.01$) increase in liver iron of Triapine-treated mice versus controls (Table 3.5). There was also a significant ($p < 0.05$) decrease of brain iron in Triapine-treated mice versus controls. A significant ($p < 0.05$) increase in splenic iron was found in mice treated with Dp44mT (0.75mg/kg/day) compared with the control (Table 3.5).

In long-term studies, there was a significant ($p < 0.05$) decrease in liver iron and a significant increase of heart iron in Dp44mT-treated mice compared to controls (Table 3.6). Interestingly, as found in short-term experiments (Table 3.5), there was a slight but not significant increase in tumour iron comparing mice treated with Dp44mT and the control in long-term studies (Table 3.6).

Table 3.5 Tissue iron levels (µg/g of tissue) of mice following treatment with vehicle control, Dp44mT or Triapine, as measured by ICP-AES in mice bearing human DMS-53 lung carcinoma xenografts treated for 2 weeks.

	Experimental Groups[a]		
	Control	*Dp44mT (0.75 mg/kg/day)*	*Triapine (12 mg/kg/day)*
Liver	579 ± 56	685 ± 74	1071 ± 162[b]
Spleen	2345 ± 339	4105 ± 402[c]	1902 ± 138
Kidney	310 ± 21	326 ± 10	293 ± 18
Heart	478 ± 26	452 ± 33	423 ± 25
Brain	114 ± 24	102 ± 13	69 ± 9[c]
Tumour	170 ± 24	373 ± 159	237 ± 57

[a] Results expressed as mean ± SEM for 12 mice.

[b] $p < 0.004$ as compared to control.

[c] $p < 0.03$ as compared to control.

Table 3.6 Tissue iron levels (µg/g of tissue) of mice following treatment with vehicle control or Dp44mT, as measured by ICP-AES in mice bearing human SK-Mel-28 melanoma xenografts treated for 7 weeks.

Organ	Experimental Groups[a]	
	Control	Dp44mT (0.4 mg/kg/day)
Liver	815 ± 50 (5)	612 ± 32 (4)[b]
Spleen	5282 ± 606 (5)	5252 ± 534 (4)
Kidney	322 ± 21 (5)	307 ± 10 (4)
Heart	437 ± 45 (5)	847 ± 11 (4)[b]
Brain	94 ± 4 (5)	81 ± 4 (4)
Tumour	359 ± 77 (4)	531 ± 98 (3)

[a] Results expressed as mean ± SEM for (n) mice.

[b] $p < 0.05$ as compared to control.

3.3.8 Effects of Chelators on Tissue Histology and Blood Cell Morphology

After a 2-week treatment period with Triapine there were increased haematopoietic cells in the splenic red pulp compared with controls in hematoxylin and eosin-stained sections (asterisks; Figures 3.4Ci and Ai, respectively). Prussian blue staining of the spleen showed that compared with the control (Figure 3.4Aii), there was increased red pulp staining (consistent with haemosiderin) in Dp44mT- and Triapine-treated mice (asterisks; Figures 3.4Bii and Cii, respectively). No splenic abnormalities were detected in mice bearing SK-Mel-28 xenografts after 7 weeks of therapy with Dp44mT (0.4 mg/kg/day) (data not shown).

In the 2-week studies, myocardial lesions were found only in Dp44mT-treated mice (arrows; Figure 3.4Biii). Such lesions consisted of poorly differentiated foci of necrosis, being replaced with immature fibrous tissue revealed by Gomori-Trichrome stain (arrows; Figure 3.4Biii). Lesion severity was dose-dependent and was more marked at higher Dp44mT doses (0.75 mg/kg/day) than at lower doses (0.4 mg/kg/day). Because the lesions are fibrotic scar tissue, they are not reversible upon drug withdrawal. After 7 weeks of Dp44mT (0.4 mg/kg/day) treatment, some myocardial fibrosis was evident (data not shown), but it was not as pronounced as that at 0.75 mg/kg/day over 2 weeks.

Liver sections stained with hematoxylin and eosin from mice treated over 2 weeks with Triapine demonstrated the presence of haematopoietic cells, present as either individual cells or small groups (arrows; Figure 3.4Civ). Accompanying this change, there was a mild increase in Kupffer cell haemosiderin in the Triapine group as shown by Prussian blue staining (arrows; Figure 4Cv). No change in liver histology was observed after a 7-week treatment with Dp44mT (0.4 mg/kg/day; data not shown).

May-Grünwald/Giemsa-stained blood smears from mice demonstrated increased anisocytosis and polychromasia in only the Triapine-treated mice after 2 weeks (data not shown). Histological assessment of tumours from 2- and 7-week treatment groups indicated increased necrosis in chelator-treated mice compared to controls (data not shown). No morphological alterations were observed in the brain or kidney over 2- or 7-weeks with any of the chelator doses (data not shown).

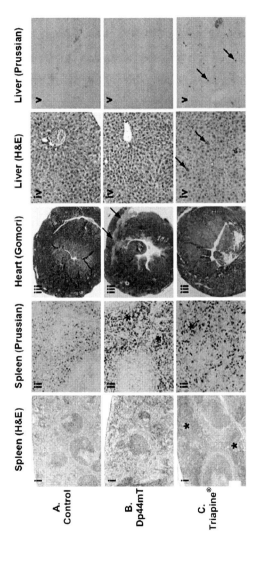

Figure 3.4 Effect of Dp44mT and Triapine on spleen, heart and liver histology from nude mice bearing DMS-53 lung carcinoma xenografts and treated i.v. with (A) control, (B) Dp44mT (0.75 mg/kg/day) or (C) Triapine (12 mg/kg/day) once per day, 5 days/week for 2 weeks. (i) Hematoxylin & eosin-stained spleen. Asterisks denote areas of increased haematopoiesis. (Magnification x40). (ii) Prussian blue-stained spleen. Asterisks denote increased Prussian blue staining of iron(III) deposits consistent with haemosiderin. (Magnification x200). (iii) Gomori-Trichrome-stained cardiac tissue. Arrows denote areas of fibrosis. (Magnification x100). (iv) Hematoxylin & eosin-stained liver. Arrows denote clusters of hematopoietic cells. (Magnification x100). (v) Prussian blue-stained liver. Arrows denote increased iron(III) deposits consistent with haemosiderin in Kupffer cells. (Magnification x100).

3.3.9 Effect of Iron Chelation on the Expression of Iron-Responsive Genes in the Tumour and Liver

Iron is crucial for proliferation and studies *in vitro* have demonstrated that chelators up-regulate the expression of iron-responsive genes such as the *TfR1* that is involved in iron uptake, *VEGF1* which plays a role in angiogenesis, and the tumour growth and metastasis suppressor gene *NDRG1* (Le and Richardson, 2004, Richardson, 2005). To understand the molecular events that follow iron chelation, we performed RT-PCR examining the mRNA expression of *NDRG1*, *TfR1* and *VEGF1* in the liver (Figure 3.5A) and tumour (Figure 3.5B). This was done in mice bearing DMS-53 tumour xenografts after short-term treatment with vehicle only, Dp44mT (0.75 mg/kg/day) or Triapine (12 mg/kg/day).

A significant decrease in the expression of *NDRG1*, *TfR1* and *VEGF1* in the liver was noted for Dp44mT- and Triapine-treated animals (Figure 3.5A). The decreased expression could be related to the increased liver iron in both Dp44mT- and Triapine-treated mice (Table 3.5). In contrast, the expression of *NDRG1*, *TfR1* and *VEGF1* mRNA was significantly increased in the tumour (Figure 3.5B). This observation was surprising considering there was no decrease in tumour iron observed in mice treated with chelators (Table 3.5). This finding could be explained by chelator-mediated changes in intracellular iron distribution that deprive the metal from certain compartments that control gene expression. Alternatively, *NDRG1*, *VEGF1* and *TfR1* are known to be regulated by the redox-sensitive transcription factor, hypoxia inducible factor-1 (HIF-1) (Le and Richardson, 2002, Le and Richardson, 2004). HIF is composed of a constitutively expressed β-subunit and an α-subunit regulated by hypoxia or iron (Le and Richardson, 2002). HIF-1α is regulated by prolyl hydroxylase; in the absence of iron or oxygen, this enzyme is inactive, preventing binding by the von Hippel-Lindau protein and inhibiting its degradation by the proteasome (Le and Richardson, 2002). Previous studies showed that increased ROS can activate HIF-1α (Chandel et al., 2000, Park et al., 2003). Because the Dp44mT-iron complex is highly-redox active (Richardson et al., 2006, Yuan et al., 2004), it can be speculated that ROS generation by this compound leads to transcription of these genes *via* HIF-1.

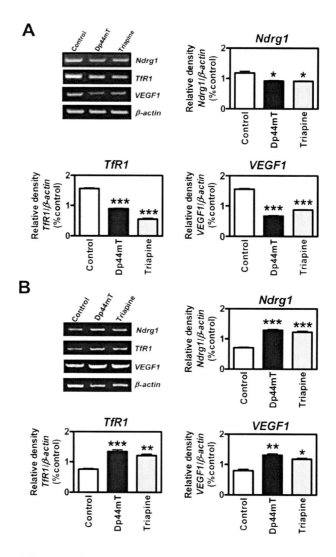

Figure 3.5 Administration of Dp44mT and Triapine to mice up-regulates the growth and metastasis suppressor, *Ndrg1* in tumour xenografts but not the liver. Expression of the iron-regulated genes *Ndrg1*, *TfR1*, and *VEGF1* is down-regulated in the (A) liver, and (B) up-regulated in the tumour, after treatment of nude mice bearing DMS-53 xenografts with Dp44mT (0.75 mg/kg/day) or Triapine (12 mg/kg/day) once per day, 5 days/week for 2 weeks. The densitometric results are mean ± SD from 3 experiments. * $p < 0.05$; ** $p < 0.01$; *** $p < 0.001$.

3.4 DISCUSSION

The development of multi-drug resistance has become a significant obstruction in the treatment of cancer (Schneider 1994). Therefore, it is necessary to develop new chemotherapeutics. For many years, the nutrient folate was targeted for anti-tumour drug development and resulted in the generation of highly successful therapeutics such as methotrexate which prevents DNA synthesis. In contrast, strategies to target iron for anti-tumour therapy have not been carefully and systematically explored. The present investigation was the first to conclusively demonstrate the marked anti-tumour efficacy of the novel iron-chelating agent Dp44mT against a range of human tumours *in vivo*.

3.4.1 *In Vitro* Evaluation

This study shows the anti-proliferative activity of the nine most effective DpT and PKIH chelators against 28 tumour lines (Table 3.2). These results *in vitro* demonstrate their broad spectrum of activity and marked anti-proliferative efficacy, with Dp44mT being particularly effective. Comparing average IC_{50} values over the 28 cell lines, we observed that Dp44mT was 21 times more effective than DOX and 47 times more efficient than Triapine (Table 3.2).

The anti-tumour efficacy of Dp44mT and the related DpT chelators has previously been shown to be due to their ability to bind cellular iron (Yuan et al., 2004). In fact, synthesis of a DpT analogue (known as Dp2mT), where the iron-binding site is completely inactivated by methylation,

87

prevented the ability of the compound to bind iron and induce anti-tumour activity (Yuan et al., 2004).

The marked activity of the DpT ligands is, in part, probably attributable to their lipophilicity, allowing them to permeate cell membranes and bind iron pools more readily than less lipid-soluble chelators *e.g.*, DFO (Richardson et al., 1995). Further, upon DpT and PKIH ligands forming iron complexes, these ligands generate cytotoxic ROS (Bernhardt et al., 2003, Chaston et al., 2004, Richardson et al., 2006, Yuan et al., 2004). The resulting oxidative damage potentiates the anti-proliferative activity of DpT and PKIH chelators compared with 311 or DFO, which bind iron but do not redox cycle (Richardson and Bernhardt, 1999). The higher activity of the DpT series relative to the PKIH class can be ascribed, at least in part, to the electrochemical potentials of their iron complexes (Bernhardt et al., 2003, Richardson et al., 2006). In fact, the $Fe^{III/II}$ redox potentials of the $Fe(DpT)_2$ complexes (+153-225 mV) are much lower than the PKIH analogues (approximately +500 mV) and lie within a range accessible to cellular oxidants and reductants (Bernhardt et al., 2003, Richardson et al., 2006).

The emergence of drug resistant tumours remains a key chemotherapeutic problem (Aouali et al., 2005). Attempts to reverse multi-drug resistance by using multi-drug resistance modulators have not yet generated optimal results (Aouali et al., 2005). Considering this, etoposide and vinblastine resistance in tumour cells did not suppress the anti-proliferative activity of Dp44mT (Figures 3.2B and C). Hence, Dp44mT may not be a substrate of ABC transporters such as P-glycoprotein and multi-drug resistant-associated protein 1, which confer resistance to vinblastine (Akiyama et al., 1985) and etoposide (Yang et al., 2005), respectively. Clearly, the ability to overcome tumour resistance to established chemotherapeutics is an important advantage of Dp44mT.

88

Because of the role of p53 in cellular arrest and apoptosis, it was vital to assess the impact of p53 on chelator anti-proliferative activity. Indeed, p53 mutations often result in a less favourable response to chemotherapy (Guimaraes and Hainaut, 2002, Lowe, 1995, O'Connor et al., 1997). In this study, p53 status did not affect the activity of DpT analogue activity, indicating a p53-independent mechanism of anti-proliferative activity, supporting their potential..

3.4.2 *In Vivo* Evaluation

This is the first study to examine the effect of Dp44mT on human tumour xenografts and to show its broad spectrum of activity *in vivo*. We demonstrate that the anti-tumour activity of Dp44mT was far greater than Triapine. For instance, in 2 week studies, Dp44mT (0.75 mg/kg/day) at a 16-fold lower dose inhibited the growth of DMS-53 xenografts more profoundly than Triapine (12 mg/kg/day; Figure 3.3A). The striking anti-tumour activity of Dp44mT (0.75 mg/kg/day) in short-term experiments using melanoma cells (Figure 3.3C) was sustained when treatment was extended to 7 weeks using 0.4 mg/kg/day (Figure 3.3D). Moreover, at the lower Dp44mT dose, cardiotoxicity was less marked.

It is significant that *in vivo*, Dp44mT did not lead to marked iron depletion of the tumour. This finding suggests that it is the effect of the chelator entering the cancer cell, binding iron, and forming the cytotoxic iron complex (Richardson et al., 2006, Yuan et al., 2004) that leads to its anti-tumour activity. In fact, we have shown that the anti-tumour efficacy of DpT chelators is proportional to their effective redox activity (Richardson et al., 2006).

The anti-tumour activity of Dp44mT in short- and long-term studies was accompanied by little alteration in normal haematological and serum biochemical indices. The lack of a pronounced effect on haematological parameters *e.g.*, RBC numbers, could be explained by the low chelator dose (0.4-0.75 mg/kg/day) required to induce anti-tumour activity. A marked increase in splenic iron after Dp44mT treatment (Table 3.5) that was confirmed by Prussian blue staining (Figure 3.4Bii) could be related to increased RBC turnover. However, there was no change in haematological indices or splenic weight in these mice. Importantly, lower Dp44mT doses (0.4 mg/kg/day) over 7 weeks, which showed marked anti-tumour activity had little effect on haematological indices (Table 3.4) or splenic iron levels (Table 3.6).

In contrast to the observations with Dp44mT, more marked alterations in haematology were observed with Triapine (12 mg/kg/day). Evidence from histology, blood smears, and haematological indices of Triapine-treated mice (Figure 3.4 and Table 3.3) indicated haematological toxicity, due to the high doses required to achieve anti-tumour activity. The pronounced increase in splenic erythropoiesis probably accounts for the rise in splenic weight in Triapine-treated mice. Our findings of haematological toxicity, together with evidence of anaemia and met-haemoglobinemia in patients treated with Triapine (Kalinowski and Richardson, 2005), draw caution to claims that Triapine is a cytoprotectant (Jiang et al., 2006).

One observation that requires note is the cardiac fibrosis observed in mice treated with the higher Dp44mT dose (0.75 mg/kg/day; Figure 3.4Biii). This effect may be due to the marked redox activity of the Dp44mT-Fe complex (Guimaraes and Hainaut, 2002, Yuan et al., 2004), as cardiotoxicity is similarly observed with anthracyclines, which may induce this effect by ROS generation (Xu et al., 2005). Such damage may be avoided by co-administering Dp44mT with suitable chelators, such as ICRF-187 (dexrazoxane) (Hasinoff et al., 2003) or DFO (Saad et al., 2001), or appropriate ROS scavengers. Here we show that cardiotoxicity of Dp44mT was dose-dependent. Hence further optimisation of the dose, administration route, and use of agents such as dexrazoxane, will be required to prevent this side effect.

The ability of chelators to up-regulate the tumour growth and metastasis suppressor, *NDRG1* (Bandyopadhyay et al., 2003, Kurdistani et al., 1998, Le and Richardson, 2004), could be vital for their anti-cancer efficacy. Our results showed that Dp44mT down-regulated these genes in mouse liver (Figure 3.5A), but caused up-regulation in tumour xenografts (Figure 3.5B). Hence, up-regulation of *NDRG1* in tumours by Dp44mT may be important for understanding its selective anti-cancer activity.

It has been suggested that up-regulation of *TfR1* and *VEGF1* by chelators may enhance tumour growth via increased iron uptake and angiogenesis, respectively (Linden and Wenger, 2003). However, their growth-promoting effects are probably overwhelmed by the chelator-mediated inhibition of ribonucleotide reductase (Green et al., 2001) and the up-regulation of *NDRG1* and other molecules, because chelators markedly inhibit tumour growth (Finch et al., 2000, Yuan et al., 2004). This principle has also been observed with the chelator desferri-exochelin (Chong et al., 2002). This ligand increased expression of the pro-apoptotic protein Nip1 and also VEGF1, but inhibited proliferation (Chong et al., 2002). The effects of chelators at inhibiting tumour growth are probably mediated through their action on many unique molecular targets (*e.g.*, ribonucleotide reductase, cyclin D1, Nip1 etc) (Abeysinghe et al., 2001, Chong et al., 2002, Gao and Richardson, 2001) and cannot be explained only by increased *NRDG1*.

In conclusion, this study demonstrates the *in vivo* efficacy of Dp44mT at inhibiting a range of human tumours. In 2-week studies, the efficacy of Dp44mT (0.75 mg/kg/day) was similar or greater than a 16-fold-greater dose of Triapine in a number of human tumour xenografts. At 0.4 mg/kg/day over 7 weeks, Dp44mT markedly inhibited melanoma growth and was well tolerated. Dp44mT caused *NDRG1* up-regulation in the tumour but not the liver, indicating a potential mechanism of selective anti-cancer activity.

CHAPTER 4

CONDITIONAL FRATAXIN KNOCKOUT IN THE FRIEDREICH'S ATAXIA HEART: TREATMENT BY IRON CHELATION THERAPY AND ELUCIDATION OF MITOCHONDRIAL IRON LOADING PATHWAYS

THIS CHAPTER CONTAINS WORK PUBLISHED IN:

Whitnall M, Rahmanto YS, Sutak R, Xu X, Becker EM, Mikhael M, Ponka P and Richardson DR (2008) The MCK mouse heart model of Friedreich's ataxia: Alterations in iron-regulated proteins and cardiac hypertrophy are limited by iron chelation. *Proc Natl Acad Sci USA* 105(28):9757-62.

4.1 INTRODUCTION

Friedreich's ataxia (FA) is the most common autosomal recessive neuro- and cardio-degenerative disorder, resulting from insufficient expression of the mitochondrial protein, frataxin (Campuzano et al., 1996). Many studies infer a role for frataxin in mitochondrial iron metabolism, particularly ISC biosynthesis (Babcock et al., 1997, Rötig et al., 1997). Deletion of the yeast frataxin homologue 1 gene, *Yfh1*, or loss of frataxin in FA patients or frataxin knockout mice, promotes mitochondrial iron accumulation, hypersensitivity to oxidants and the loss of mitochondrial DNA and ISC-containing enzymes (Babcock et al., 1997, Puccio et al., 2001, Rötig et al., 1997, Wilson and Roof, 1997). Increased cardiac iron deposition and perturbations in haem biosynthesis and ATP production suggest FA pathogenesis is linked to mitochondrial iron overload (Richardson, 2003). Furthermore, the anti-oxidant idebenone, improves heart and neurological function in FA patients, suggesting the presence of oxidant stress (Rustin et al., 1999).

Iron loading can lead to toxicity in iron overload disease due to the ability of iron to redox cycle, leading to cytotoxic radicals (Richardson, 2003). The potential of iron loading to become toxic may be more pronounced in the highly redox-active mitochondrial environment (Rötig et al., 1997). There is no effective treatment for FA, although evidence of mitochondrial iron loading within cardiomyocytes from FA patients supports the use of chelation as a therapeutic strategy (Richardson, 2003). The iron chelator DFO, has some ability to rescue FA fibroblasts from oxidant stress (Wong et al., 1999). However, the inability of DFO to permeate the mitochondrion means it is ineffective for FA treatment (Richardson, 2003, Richardson et al., 2001).

To circumvent the poor permeability of DFO (Richardson, 2003), the lipophilic, membrane-permeable chelator, PIH, which mobilises mitochondrial iron (Richardson et al., 2001), was developed (Richardson and Ponka, 1998). Studies *in vitro*, *in vivo* and in a clinical trial have shown the marked chelation efficacy and high tolerability of PIH (Richardson, 2003, Richardson et al., 2001, Richardson and Ponka, 1998, Wong et al., 2004).

Cardiomyopathy is a frequent cause of death in FA (Delatycki et al., 2000). To test the potential of iron chelation therapy for FA treatment, the muscle creatine kinase conditional frataxin knockout mouse was used (Puccio et al., 2001). This model lacks frataxin in cardiomyocytes and exhibits classical phenotypic traits of the cardiomyopathy in FA, including marked cardiac mitochondrial iron accumulation and deficiency in ISC enzymes (Puccio et al., 2001).

In this section of work it is demonstrated that frataxin deficiency leads to abnormal iron metabolism *in vivo* in MCK mutant mice, and that treatment with PIH and DFO prevents cardiac iron loading and limits myocardial hypertrophy.

4.2 MATERIALS AND METHODS

4.2.1 Animals

Using a conditional gene-targeting approach, frataxin knockout (mutant) and wild-type (WT) mice were generated by and obtained from Dr Hélène Puccio and Prof. Michel Koenig (Institut de Génétique et de Biologie Moléculaire et Cellulaire, Université Louis Pasteur, Strasbourg, France). These mice carry a tissue-specific Cre transgene under the control of the muscle creatine kinase (MCK) promoter, that induces deletion of *Frda* exon 4 (encoding the protein, frataxin) from cardiac and skeletal muscle only (Puccio et al., 2001). The frataxin deficient mouse (MCK mutant) very closely mimics the important pathophysiological and biochemical features associated with FA in humans, including cardiac hypertrophy and mitochondrial iron loading (Puccio et al., 2001).

4.2.2 Genotyping

Male and female MCK mutant and WT mice were genotyped using genomic tail DNA and multiplex PCR *via* standard techniques (Puccio et al., 2001). Briefly, 3-week-old MCK mice were tail-tipped (approximately 5 mm of tail per mouse) and the tail tip placed in sterile tubes. Tail tips were dissolved overnight at 65 °C. Genomic DNA was isolated and purified for PCR analysis using the ABI Prism™ 6100 Nucleic Acid Prepstation (Applied Biosystems, Melbourne, Australia) in accordance with the protocol provided by the manufacturer (Applied Biosystems).

Using the specific primer pairs listed in Table 4.1 (Puccio et al., 2001), PCR amplification was performed under the following conditions. The

PCR reaction mixture contained 200 µM of each dNTP, 1.0 µM of each primer, 1.5 mM MgCl2, 1x PCR Buffer II and 1.0 U AmpliTaq® DNA polymerase (Applied Biosystems). PCR cycles were performed on a DNA Engine PTC-200 Peltier Thermal Cycler (BioRad) and consisted of 3 min at 94 °C (initial denaturation), followed by 40 cycles at 94 °C for 45 sec (denaturation), 61 °C for 45 sec (annealing) and 72 °C for 1 min (extension), with a single final extension period of 10 min at 72 °C. The PCR products were separated *via* electrophoresis on a 1.5% agarose gel in 1x TAE buffer and visualised with EtBr staining. DNA size standards (Promega) were run on each gel.

Table 4.1 Sequences of primers used to amplify MCK tail DNA.

Pair No.	Primer name	Oligonucleotides (5'-3')		Product size (bp)
		Forward	Reverse	
1	*Frataxin WT*	CTGTTTACCATGGCT GAGATCTC	CCAAGGATATAACAG ACACCATT	500
2	*Frataxin KO*	CTGTTTACCATGGCT GAGATCTC	CGCCTCCCCTACCCG GTAGATTC	250

4.2.3 Chelator Studies

PIH was synthesised as previously described (Richardson and Ponka, 1998) and DFO was purchased from Novartis. Chelators were dissolved in a vehicle solution of 20% propylene glycol in 0.9% saline at a concentration of 150 mg/kg. Treatment *via* intraperitoneal (i.p.) injection with vehicle alone or vehicle containing DFO and PIH, commenced when mice were 4.5

weeks of age and continued over 5 consecutive days per week until mice were 8.5 weeks of age.

After this time, mice were sacrificed (Section 2.2.2), organ weights assessed (Section 2.2.2) and blood taken for haematological analysis as per Sections 2.3.1. Harvested tissues were used for histochemistry (Section 2.3.3), measurement of tissue iron stores (Section 2.3.2), IRP-RNA binding activity assays (Section 2.6) and RT-PCR and western analysis as below. Image analysis was performed using Zeiss KS-400 software (Carl Zeiss, Munich, Germany) to quantitate Prussian blue stained sections.

4.2.4 RT-PCR Analysis

RNA was isolated from heart tissue as described in Section 2.4.1. RT-PCR was performed by Dr Yohan Suryo Rahmanto (Iron Metabolism and Chelation lab, University of Sydney) as per section 2.4.2, using the primers in Table 4.2. Densitometric analysis was performed as per Section 2.8.1.

Table 4.2 Sequences and accession numbers of primers used to amplify RNA extracted from heart tissue.

Primer name	Accession no.	Oligonucleotides (5'-3')		Product size (bp)
		Forward	Reverse	
Frataxin	NM_008044	GCCACGCCCATT TGAACC	GCCGCTGGAAGGA GAAGA	326
TfR1	NM_011638	TCCCGAGGGTTA TGTGGC	GGCGGAAACTGAG TATGATTGA	324
H-Ferritin	NM_010239	TTTGACCGAGAT GATGTG	TCAGTAGCCAGTTT GTGC	248
L-Ferritin	NM_008049	TGGCTCTGGAAG GGCGTAG	GGTTGCCCATCTTC TTGAT	315

Ferroportin 1	NM_016917	AACATCCGTGAA CTTGAA	CCATTGATAATGCC TCTTT	665
MIT Ferritin	NM_026286	CCAGGTATCCTTT AGGTCC	AGGCCAGAGTATG TAAGTCC	432
GAPDH	NM_008084	ATTCAACGGCAC AGTCAA	CTTCTGGGTGGCAG TGAT	394

4.2.5 Western Analysis

Protein was isolated from heart tissue as described in Section 2.5.1. Western blot analysis was performed as per Section 2.5.2, using antibodies against ferroportin1 (Dr. David Haile, University Texas Health Science Center, San Antonio, USA) at a dilution of 1:2500, frataxin (US Biologicals, Swampscott, USA) at 1:1000, H-, L- and MIT ferritin (Prof. Sonia Levi, San Raffaele Institute, Milan, Italy) at 1:1000, TfR1 (Invitrogen) at 1:4000, and succinate dehydrogenase complex subunit A (SDHA; Santa Cruz Biotechnology) at 1:500. Additionally, the internal control, GAPDH (Santa Cruz Biotechnology) was used at a dilution of 1:2000. Densitometric analysis was performed as per Section 2.8.1

4.2.6 Uptake and Intracellular Distribution of [59]Fe *In Vivo*

MCK mutant and WT mice were i.v. injected with ^{59}Fe-Tf as per Section 2.7. Mice were sacrificed 24 h post i.v. injection of ^{59}Fe-Tf and the hearts removed and washed as per Section 2.7. Radioactivity of ^{59}Fe in whole hearts was measured using a Wallac WIZARD 1480 γ-counter (PerkinElmer) to assess ^{59}Fe uptake into the heart.

Subsequently, to measure the intracellular distribution of ^{59}Fe in the heart samples, cytosolic and stromal mitochondrial membrane (SMM) fractions were prepared using the methods outlined in Section 2.7. Additionally, the SMM pellet was resuspended in ice-cold ST buffer containing 1.5% Triton X-100 and centrifuged at 16, 000 g/45 min/4 °C to remove any insoluble material (pellet) from the soluble SMM (supernatant). Radioactivity of ^{59}Fe in the cytosolic and soluble SMM fractions was measured using a Wallac WIZARD 1480 γ-counter.

4.2.7 Native PAGE ^{59}Fe Autoradiography and Anion-Exchange Chromatography

MCK mutant and WT mice were i.v. injected with ^{59}Fe-Tf as per Section 2.7. Mice were sacrificed 2-96 h post i.v. injection of ^{59}Fe-Tf, the hearts removed and washed, and cytosolic fractions prepared (Section 2.7). Radioactivity was measured using a Wallac WIZARD 1480 γ-counter and cytosolic fractions then used for either native gradient PAGE ^{59}Fe autoradiography or anion-exchange chromatography, performed by Dr Robert Sutak and Shawn Xu (Iron Metabolism and Chelation lab), as below.

Cytosolic lysates were prepared, separated using 3-12% native gradient PAGE gels and the resulting ^{59}Fe distribution assessed using autoradiography, all according to established techniques (Richardson et al., 1996, Wong et al., 2004). Densitometric analysis was performed using software described in Section 2.8.1. Additionally, cytosolic samples were also incubated for 1 h with anti-H- and L-ferritin antibodies (Section 4.2.5) to perform supershifts *via* native gradient PAGE ^{59}Fe autoradiography (Richardson et al., 1996, Wong et al., 2004).

Cytosolic lysates were prepared and anion-exchange chromatography performed using established protocols (Babusiak et al., 2005). Briefly, samples were loaded onto a Mono Q 5/50 GL column (Amersham Biosciences) and fractions eluted with 20 mM HEPES (pH 8.0) and linear gradient of 0-1 M NaCl using a BioLogic Duo Flow Fast Pressure Liquid Chromatography system (BioRad). The ^{59}Fe in eluted fractions was measured using a Wallac WIZARD 1480 γ-counter.

4.3 RESULTS

4.3.1 Altered Cardiac Iron Metabolism in the Mutant

Little is known regarding the function of frataxin *in vivo* and the role of iron loading in FA pathogenesis. To this end, the metabolism of iron in MCK mutants and the potential of iron chelation to prevent cardiomyopathy, were examined. This model was chosen as it closely reflects the alterations in the heart of FA patients, including mitochondrial iron loading (Puccio et al., 2001). The iron accumulation is observed only after 7 weeks of age with no detectable deposits being found earlier (Puccio et al., 2001).

In initial studies, cardiac iron uptake was assessed using the physiological serum iron binding protein ^{59}Fe-Tf to radio-label 9-week-old WT and mutant mice *via* i.v. tail vein injection. Incorporation of ^{59}Fe into the whole heart was measured after 24 h. A significant ($p < 0.001$) increase in the level of cardiac ^{59}Fe was observed in mutant mice compared to WT controls (Figure 4.1A). To assess the intracellular distribution of ^{59}Fe, hearts were fractionated to yield cytosolic and SMM fractions. It was evident in mutant compared to WT mice that there was a marked decrease in the proportion of cytosolic ^{59}Fe, although there was a significant ($p <$ 0.001) increase of ^{59}Fe in the SMM (Figure 4.1B). This result directly confirmed that deletion of frataxin leads to mitochondrial iron loading in the mutant (Puccio et al., 2001) and results in a relative cytosolic iron deficiency.

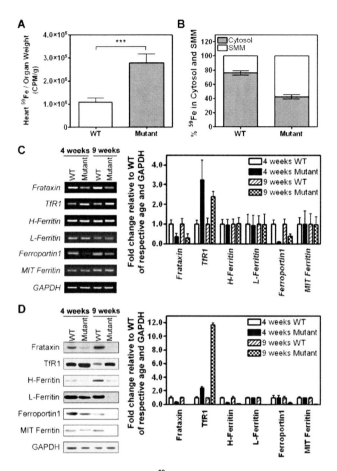

Figure 4.1 Marked alterations in ^{59}Fe uptake, distribution and expression of molecules that play key roles in iron metabolism occur in mutant relative to WT mice. (A) Iron uptake from ^{59}Fe-Tf into the heart is increased in the mutant. Mutant and WT mice (9-weeks-old) were injected i.v. with ^{59}Fe-Tf and sacrificed 24 h later. Hearts were washed and assessed for ^{59}Fe-activity. **(B) Mutant hearts show a cytosolic iron deficiency relative to the stromal-mitochondrial membrane (SMM).** Hearts from (A) were processed as described in the *Materials and Methods* and the cytosol and SMM separated and assessed for ^{59}Fe activity. **(C, D) Examination of (C) mRNA and (D) protein expression of frataxin and molecules involved in iron metabolism in hearts from 4- and 9-week-old WT and mutant mice.** mRNA and protein expression were assessed as per *Materials and Methods*. Densitometry is expressed relative to the respective WT at each age and GAPDH. Results in A and B are mean ± SD (3 experiments). The RT-PCR and Western panels in C and D are typical experiments, while the densitometry is mean ± SD (3-5 experiments). *** p < 0.001.

103

Considering the alterations in ^{59}Fe uptake and distribution, the changes that occur at the mRNA and protein levels of molecules which are involved in cardiac iron metabolism were examined, comparing WT and mutant mice at both 4 and 9 weeks of age. These ages were chosen because at 4 weeks, no overt phenotype was present, whereas at 9 weeks, a severe cardiomyopathy was found (Puccio et al., 2001). There was a significant ($p < 0.001$) decrease in frataxin expression at the mRNA (Figure 4.1C) and protein levels (Figure 4.1D) in 4- and 9-week-old mutants. However, frataxin expression was not totally ablated, due to other cells within the total heart homogenate apart from cardiomyocytes (*e.g.*, fibroblasts), which are not targeted by the conditional knockout strategy (Puccio et al., 2001).

TfR1 was significantly ($p < 0.001$) up-regulated in 4- and 9-week-old mutants relative to WT mice at the mRNA (Figure4. 1C) and protein (Figure 4.1D) levels. The extent of TfR1 protein up-regulation in mutants was significantly ($p < 0.001$) more pronounced at 9 than 4 weeks of age (Figure 4.1D).

The iron-storage protein ferritin, is composed of heavy (H) and light (L) chains (Dunn et al., 2007). Comparing WT and mutant mice at 4 and 9 weeks of age, *H-* and *L-ferritin* mRNA expression was not markedly or significantly altered (Figure 4.1C). In contrast, Western analysis showed a significant ($p < 0.001$) decrease in H- and L-ferritin protein expression in mutants compared to WT mice at 9 weeks of age (Figure 4.1D). The molecular alterations in TfR1 and ferritin expression suggest the cytosol was in an iron-deficient state. This hypothesis was supported by the significantly ($p < 0.001$) decreased expression of the iron export molecule ferroportin1, in mutant compared to WT mice at the mRNA and protein levels at 9 weeks of age (Figures 4.1C and 4.1D). Because ferroportin1 protein expression is down-regulated by decreased cellular iron levels (Lymboussaki et al., 2003), this further supports the idea that cardiomyocytes are experiencing a cytosolic iron deficiency.

Mitochondrial (MIT) ferritin is thought to act as an iron-storage protein within this organelle (Levi et al., 2001). Similarly to cytosolic H- and L-ferritin expression, there was no alteration in *MIT ferritin* mRNA between mutant and WT mice at both ages (Figure 4.1C), although a decrease in protein expression was detected in mutant mice, particularly at 9 weeks of age (Figure 4.1D). It is notable that to detect this mRNA, 40 cycles of PCR were necessary in both genotypes, suggesting it was very poorly expressed. This observation suggested MIT ferritin was not playing a role in storing iron in the mutant, as a marked increase in its expression would be expected to accommodate the iron loading.

The observations above indicate pronounced alterations in cardiac iron homeostasis caused by deletion of frataxin. Given that IRP1 and IRP2 are key regulators of TfR1, ferritin and ferroportin1 expression (Dunn et al., 2007), we examined IRP-RNA binding activity in mutant and WT mice.

4.3.2 IRP2-RNA Binding Activity is Increased in Mutant Heart

Iron metabolism is regulated, in part, by IRP1 and IRP2, which interact with iron-response elements (IREs) in the 3' untranslated region (UTR) of *TfR1* mRNA or 5' UTR of *H-* and *L-ferritin* or *ferroportin1* mRNA, in response to cytosolic iron (Dunn et al., 2007). IRP-binding to the 3' UTR IRE stabilizes *TfR1* mRNA, increasing its expression, while binding to the 5' IREs of *ferritin* or *ferroportin1* mRNA inhibits translation (Dunn et al., 2007, Meyron-Holtz et al., 2004a, Meyron-Holtz et al., 2004b).

Gel-retardation analysis indicated significantly ($p < 0.01$) increased IRP2-RNA binding activity in mutant relative to WT mice only at 9 weeks of age, while there was little alteration in IRP1-RNA binding (Figure 4.2). It has been demonstrated that β-mercaptoethanol (β-ME) converts IRP1 to its RNA-binding state (Meyron-Holtz et al., 2004a, Meyron-Holtz et al., 2004b). However, its addition to lysates did not significantly increase IRP1-binding activity (Figure 4.2). This indicated that IRP1 was largely in its active RNA binding form in WT and mutant mice at 4 and 9 weeks of age.

Previous studies indicated IRP2 is crucial in controlling iron-regulated gene expression *in vivo* at physiological oxygen tension (Meyron-Holtz et al., 2004a, Meyron-Holtz et al., 2004b). This is because in contrast to IRP1, only IRP2 registers intracellular iron levels and modulates its RNA binding activity at physiological oxygen levels (Meyron-Holtz et al., 2004a, Meyron-Holtz et al., 2004b). Indeed, our results are consistent with the theory of Rouault and colleagues (Meyron-Holtz et al., 2004a, Meyron-Holtz et al., 2004b), that IRP2 primarily regulates mammalian iron homeostasis *in vivo* despite its lower expression compared to IRP1.

The increased IRP2 activity in 9-week-old mutants confirms a cytosolic iron deficiency, which could mediate the marked up-regulation of TfR1 and down-regulation of ferritin and ferroportin1 protein (Figure 4.1D). As there was no alteration in IRP1- or IRP2-RNA binding activity at 4-weeks of age (Figure 4.2), other factors (*e.g.*, at the transcriptional level) could be responsible for the less pronounced alteration in TfR1 and ferritin expression at this time.

106

The elevated IRP2-RNA binding activity in mutant relative to WT mice (Figure 4.2) and increased iron uptake into the heart (Figure 4.1A) and SMM (Figure 4.1B), suggest frataxin deficiency leads to a major alteration in iron trafficking. Specifically, lack of frataxin leads to a cytosolic iron deficiency relative to mitochondrial iron loading.

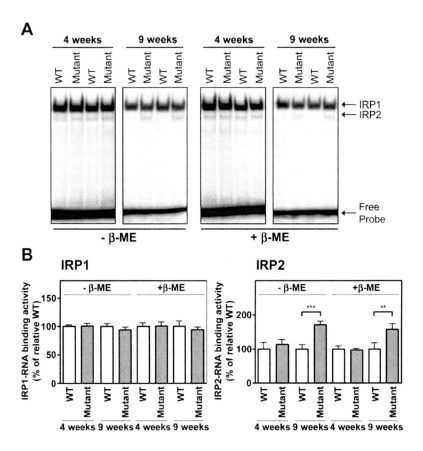

Figure 4.2 IRP2-RNA binding activity in the heart is increased in mutant mice relative to the WT at 9-weeks but not 4-weeks of age, while IRP1-RNA binding does not alter. (A, B) IRP-RNA binding activity was assayed by gel-retardation analysis. At 4- and 9-weeks of age WT and mutant mice were sacrificed, the heart washed and homogenized in Munro buffer. Equal amounts of heart extract were assayed in the absence and presence of β-mercaptoethanol (β-ME). Results in **(A)** are from a typical experiment, while the densitometry in **(B)** is mean ± SD of 3 experiments.

** $p < 0.01$; *** $p < 0.001$.

4.3.3 Marked Alterations in Cytosolic ^{59}Fe Distribution within Ferritin in Mutant Heart

To directly assess the altered distribution of cardiac iron within subcellular compartments, 9-week-old WT and mutant mice were radio-labelled *via* injection of ^{59}Fe-Tf and then sacrificed 2-96 h later. The cytosol was extracted from whole heart and separated using 3-12% native gradient PAGE and ^{59}Fe distribution assessed by autoradiography (Figure 4.3A).

A clear difference in the cytosolic ^{59}Fe distribution was found in mutants compared to their WT counterparts at all time points (Figure 4.3A). In the cytosol of WT mice, a major ^{59}Fe-containing band (band A) and a smaller more diffuse band (band B) were observed (Figure 4.3A). Band A co-migrated with horse spleen ferritin (data not shown). This ^{59}Fe distribution is consistent with previous studies assessing ^{59}Fe distribution in primary cultures of WT cardiomyocytes, in which ^{59}Fe-labelled ferritin was present as two bands (Wong et al., 2004). In contrast, the majority of ^{59}Fe in mutants appeared as a more faint and smeared band (band C Figure 4.3A). We showed that bands A, B and C correspond to ^{59}Fe-ferritin, as they could be supershifted with anti-H- or L-ferritin antibodies (Figure 4.3A). Control antibodies to other proteins   (*e.g.,* cyclin D1) had no effect on supershifting these bands (data not shown).

Densitometric analysis showed that ^{59}Fe-ferritin in the mutant expressed as a percentage of the WT, increased from 60% after 2 h incubation with ^{59}Fe-Tf to 74% after 4 h (Figure 4.3B). After 24-96 h incubation, cytosolic ^{59}Fe-ferritin in the mutant increased to the same level as that of the WT (Figure 4.3B). This result appears to conflict with the data in Figure 4.1B.

However, we note that the results in Figure 4.3B represent ^{59}Fe- ferritin, which is only a sub-component of the total iron shown in Figure 4.1B.

To characterise the ^{59}Fe-ferritin distribution, we performed anion exchange chromatography using cytosol from ^{59}Fe-labeled heart (Figure 4.3C). Interestingly, the WT lysate showed two major ^{59}Fe-containing peaks in fractions 14-16 and 18-20 (Figure 4.3C) that appeared to correspond to bands B and A observed after native PAGE ^{59}Fe autoradiography (Figure 4.3A). In contrast, the mutant lysate had only one major peak in fractions 14-17 (Figure 4.3C), which appeared to correspond to band C in Figure 4.3A.

Collectively, these data indicate differences exist in the molecular distribution of ^{59}Fe in ferritin of mutant compared to WT mice.

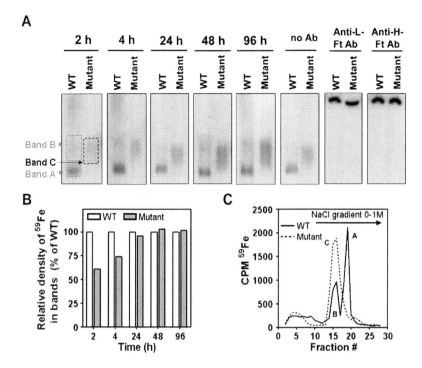

Figure 4.3 Intracellular ^{59}Fe distribution in cytosolic ferritin is markedly different in mutant mice relative to WT animals. (A) Native PAGE ^{59}Fe-autoradiography identifies 2 ^{59}Fe-containing bands in the cytosol of WT mice (band "A", "B") and 1 (band "C") in the mutant. Anti-ferritin antibody (anti-L or –H Ft) supershifts bands "A" and "B" in WT and band "C" in mutant mice. WT or mutants were injected i.v. with ^{59}Fe-Tf and sacrificed after 2-96 h. The hearts were washed, homogenized at 4°C and cytosol prepared for native PAGE-^{59}Fe-autoradiography by centrifugation at 16,500 g/45 min/4°C. Anti-L- or H-ferritin antibody was added to cytosolic lysates and incubated for 1 h at room temperature before native PAGE ^{59}Fe-autoradiography was performed. (B) Densitometry of the bands in the WT and mutant mice shown in panel A. The density of bands "A" and "B" in the WT were added and are compared to band "C" in the mutant. (C) Anion-exchange chromatography of the cytosolic fraction prepared in (A) demonstrates 2 major forms of ^{59}Fe in the WT ("A" and "B") relative to 1 major peak ("C") in the mutant. Proteins were eluted by a linear gradient of 0-1 M NaCl and ^{59}Fe measured by a γ-counter. Results are typical experiments from 3 performed.

4.3.4 Iron Chelation

Considering the potential role of mitochondrial iron accumulation in the mutant cardiomyopathy and the marked alterations in iron metabolism, experiments were initiated to assess the effect of chelation on body weight loss and cardiac hypertrophy. In these studies, PIH (150 mg/kg) (Richardson et al., 2001) was combined with the more hydrophilic DFO (150 mg/kg) (Richardson, 2003). This combination is known to increase iron mobilisation due to the ability of lipid-soluble PIH to mobilise cell iron and donate it to the largely extracellular ligand, DFO (Link et al., 2003).

Chelator treatment was initiated at 4.5 weeks-of-age, before visible signs of the disease were evident, and continued 5 days/week until animals reached 8.5 weeks of age, when the phenotype was pronounced (Puccio et al., 2001). Initially, male and female mouse data were separated due to the difference in iron metabolism between the sexes (Sproule et al., 2001). However, the results obtained for both sexes were similar and thus combined.

4.3.4.1 Chelation Reduces Heart Iron in the Mutant

Heart iron levels were significantly ($p < 0.001$) greater in mutants (462 $\pm$ 19 µg/g; $n = 27$) than in WT mice (328 $\pm$ 9 µg/g; $n = 34$) when treated with vehicle control alone (Figure 4.4A).

Treatment of mutants with PIH/DFO resulted in a significant ($p < 0.001$) decrease in cardiac iron (282 $\pm$ 13 µg/g; $n = 21$) compared to mutants treated with the vehicle at   8.5 weeks of age (Figure 4.4A). This was confirmed by Prussian blue staining which was significantly ($p < 0.001$) decreased in mutants following treatment with chelators to a level comparable to the vehicle-treated WT (Figure 4.4B). These results showed that chelators effectively decreased cardiac iron in the mutants to the level in WT mice treated with vehicle alone, but did not lead to overt cardiac iron depletion (Figures 4.4A and B). In mutant and WT mice, chelation reduced iron levels in the liver, spleen and kidney by 21-28%, 12-26% and 6-10%, respectively, of that found for the WT vehicle control. However, this reduction was only significant ($p < 0.05$) for the liver. Treatment with chelators had no effect on histology of the heart (Figure 4.4B) or any other major organs (data not shown), indicating that it was well tolerated. Assessment of haematological indices between chelator- and vehicle-treated mice showed the 4-week treatment did not lead to decreased erythrocyte count, haemoglobin concentration or haematocrit (Table 4.3).

Table 4.3. Haematological indices of mice treated with vehicle (control) or PIH/DFO.

Parameter	Experimental Group			
	Vehicle		150 mg/kg PIH/DFO	
	WT	Mutant	WT	Mutant
RBC (x 10^{12}/L)	8.3 ± 0.3 (18)	7.6 ± 0.4 (13)	8.28 ± 0.4 (16)	9.3 ± 0.4 (8)
WBC (x 10^9/L)	5.7 ± 0.5 (18)	3.5 ± 0.3 (14)	7.0 ± 0.8 (16)	6.2 ± 0.4 (8)
Hb (g/L)	152.3 ± 2.8 (17)	143.1 ± 4.0 (14)	161.6 ± 2.5 (16)	170.3 ± 7.3 (8)
Hct	0.46 ± 0.02 (18)	0.42 ± 0.03 (14)	0.47 ± 0.03 (16)	0.52 ± 0.03 (8)
Platelet (x 10^9/L)	996.3 ± 170.6 (13)	864.0 ± 151.5 (12)	1153.5 ± 111.8 (11)	882.4 ± 236.9 (5)

Data are expressed as mean ± SEM for (*n*) mice as indicated

Abbreviations: RBC, red blood cell; Hb, haemoglobin; Hct, haematocrit; WBC, white blood cell.

4.3.4.2 Growth After Chelation

The first evidence of weight loss and retarded animal growth in vehicle-treated mutants was at 6 weeks of age, as similarly reported (Puccio et al., 2001). The body weight of vehicle-treated mutants continued to decline until the study endpoint at 8.5-weeks of age (Figure 4.4C).

Treatment of WT mice with 150 mg/kg of PIH/DFO had no significant negative impact on body weight as determined through comparison to WT mice treated with vehicle alone (Figure 4.4C). These data indicated that the chelators were well tolerated. However, treatment of mutant mice with PIH/DFO did not significantly prevent the decline in body weight observed in mutants treated with vehicle from 6- to 8.5-weeks of age (Figure 4.4C). Phenotypically, chelator-treated mutants were indistinguishable from those treated with vehicle; both groups experiencing weight loss (Figure 4.4C) and adopted a hunched stance at 8.5 weeks of age (data not shown).

4.3.4.3 Chelation Limits Heart Hypertrophy

Heart weight (Figure 4.4D) and the heart to body weight ratio (Figure 4.4E) are markers of hypertrophy (Puccio et al., 2001) and were measured to assess the effects of iron chelation. The increase in heart weight and heart to body weight ratio in the mutants compared to the WT mice were clearly evident and significant ($p < 0.001$) when mice were treated with the vehicle.

In the chelator-treated mice, there was a significant ($p < 0.001$) difference between the heart weight (Figure 4.4D) and heart to body weight ratio (Figure 4.4E) in mutant and control animals. However, assessing chelator-treated mutants, there was a significant decrease in both heart weight ($p <$

0.01; Figure 4.4D) and heart to body weight ratio ($p < 0.05$; Figure 4.4E) compared to mutant mice treated with vehicle. Hence, the chelator-treatment limited the cardiomyopathy but did not totally rescue the phenotype. Indeed, echocardiography showed no difference in ventricular function between mutants treated with chelators or vehicle at 8.5 weeks of age (data not shown).

The chelator combination was well tolerated by the mice and did not have any negative effect on the heart, there being no difference in heart weight (Figure 4.4D) or heart to body weight ratios (Figure 4.4E) in WT animals treated with the vehicle alone or PIH/DFO.

The effect of chelators on rescuing the metabolic defect in FA was also examined by assessing myocardial expression of SDHA. This ISC enzyme is critical for mitochondrial energy metabolism and is markedly decreased in the mutant compared to WT (Puccio et al., 2001, Sutak et al., 2008). Examining 8.5-week-old mice treated with vehicle or PIH/DFO, it was clear the chelators did not prevent the decrease in SDHA expression (Figure 4.4F). This again confirmed chelator treatment limited cardiac hypertrophy, but could not rescue the metabolic defect. Further, in WT animals, chelator treatment was effective as it increased ($p < 0.001$) TfR1 by 225% relative to WT mice treated with vehicle (Figure 4.4F). In mutants, TfR1 expression was far greater than in the WT. However, chelator treatment in the mutant did not further increase TfR1 relative to the vehicle, probably because its expression was already very pronounced relative to that of WT mice (Figure 4.4F).

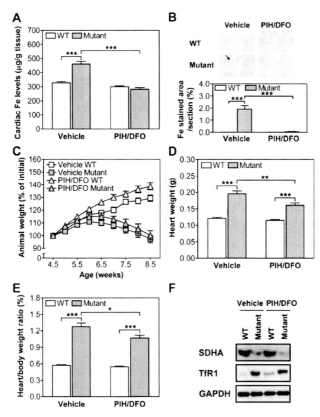

Figure 4.4 Combination of the mitochondrial-permeable chelator, PIH, with the hydrophilic ligand, DFO, prevents cardiomyocyte iron loading in the mutant and limits cardiac hypertrophy. However, it does not rescue weight loss or decreased succinate dehydrogenase (SDHA) expression in the mutant relative to WT. (A, B) PIH/DFO prevents cardiac Fe accumulation in mutants. WT and mutant mice (4.5-weeks-old) were injected i.p. with 150 mg/kg of PIH and DFO 5 days/week/4-weeks. Upon sacrifice, the heart was washed and iron measured by: **(A)** ICP-AES for total iron, or **(B)** histological quantitation of Prussian blue staining using Zeiss KS-400 software (Magnification 100x). The arrow denotes blue iron deposits in cardiomyocytes. The plot illustrates the area of blue iron deposits/section (30 sections/group; mean ± SEM). **(C) Mutant mice lose body weight irrespective of treatment with vehicle or PIH/DFO.** WT and mutants were treated as in **(A)** and their weight measured. **(D, E) PIH/DFO significantly limits cardiac hypertrophy in the mutant as measured by (D) heart weight or (E) heart to body weight ratio.** Animals were treated as in **(A)**. **(F) PIH/DFO does not prevent loss of SDHA expression in mutants, but up-regulates TfR1 in WT mice.** Mice were treated as in **(A)** and hearts used for Western analysis. Results in A, C, D and E are mean ± SEM (n = 21-35 mice). Histology in **(B)** and results in **(F)** are typical experiments from 4 performed. * $p < 0.05$; ** $p < 0.01$; *** $p < 0.001$.

4.4 DISCUSSION

At present, there is no effective treatment for the severe debilitating cardiac effects observed in FA. Considering that iron accumulation is toxic (Richardson, 2003), the discovery that mitochondrial iron accumulation occurs in frataxin knockout mice (Puccio et al., 2001) and in FA patients (Richardson, 2003), provides a potential target for therapeutic intervention.

This section of work demonstrates that iron accumulation in MCK mutants is mediated by increased iron uptake from Tf due to TfR1 up-regulation. The decreased frataxin expression leads to iron targeted to the mitochondrion and a relative cytosolic iron deficiency, low ferritin expression and decreased expression of the iron exporter, ferroportin1. Hence, frataxin deficiency leads to decreased ISC synthesis, which results in a compensatory increase in iron transport to the mitochondrion. This response may be an attempt to rescue the decreased ISC synthesis that is vital for energy generation *etc*. A model summarising the altered iron trafficking observed is presented in Figure 4.5. These alterations in iron metabolism were important to delineate, in order to understand the mechanisms responsible for the mitochondrial iron loading and, in part, the cardiac pathology observed.

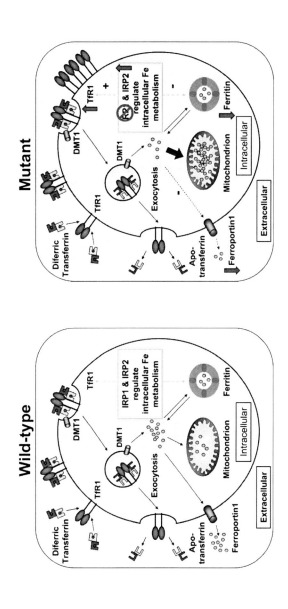

Figure 4.5 Schematic diagram of the alterations in iron trafficking in mutant compared to WT mice. Ablation of frataxin decreases ISC synthesis that is vital for energy generation. There is increased TfR1 and decreased ferritin and ferroportin1 in the mutant relative to the WT mouse. These changes are likely mediated in older mutants by increased IRP2-RNA binding.

119

Similar changes in the expression of molecules involved in the transport and storage of iron have been observed in cells hyper-expressing MIT ferritin (Nie et al., 2006, Nie et al., 2005). In this case, there was down-regulation of frataxin expression, up-regulation of TfR1, down-regulation of ferritin, cytosolic iron deficiency and mitochondrial iron overload. Furthermore, ISC synthesis and haem biogenesis were markedly reduced. This may be due to MIT ferritin sequestering iron, making it unavailable for these essential mitochondrial processes (Nie et al., 2006, Nie et al., 2005). Hence, the defect caused by forced MIT ferritin expression resembles some consequences of frataxin deficiency.

Previous data in combination with the current study indicate that a major control of iron uptake is mitochondrial iron utilisation for functions such as ISC synthesis, which is depressed in the absence of frataxin (Chen et al., 2002). The mechanism of communication between the mitochondrion and cytosol that alters iron trafficking to "satisfy" the mitochondrial demand remains unknown. However, the lack of ISC synthesis and its decreased release into the cytosol could be involved. It is relevant that mutations in *ABCB7*, which is involved in mitochondrial ISC export, results in mitochondrial iron accumulation leading to sideroblastic anaemia with ataxia (Allikmets et al., 1999). Further, it can be speculated that alterations in endosomal/organelle or iron-chaperone trafficking may be involved in directing iron targeting between the cytosol and mitochondrion. Direct endosomal and mitochondrial contact to effect mitochondrial iron targeting may occur in erythroid cells (Richardson et al., 1996, Sheftel et al., 2007). In addition, it is well known that organelle and transporter trafficking is involved in copper transport (Greenough et al., 2004). Thus, further studies are required to define the alterations in iron trafficking in the mutants.

Considering the changes in MCK mutant iron metabolism and the mitochondrial iron accumulation that could be toxic, we combined PIH and DFO to treat mice. The results in this chapter show that iron chelation prevents cardiac iron accumulation in mutants and limits cardiac hypertrophy. However, this therapy did not totally rescue the defect due to loss of frataxin, with mutants still suffering decreased cardiac function. Deterioration of mutants despite iron chelation therapy indicates chelator-insensitive or iron-independent events occur that contribute to death. Clearly, chelation cannot replace frataxin in ISC synthesis, but it may prevent the oxidative damage due to mitochondrial iron accumulation. Hence, this could explain the partial rescue observed.

It is significant that chelation prevented iron accumulation in mutants, but did not lead to overt cardiac iron depletion or toxicity. These observations have implications for FA patients. Indeed, a valid criticism against chelation therapy for FA is that it could result in whole-body iron depletion (Richardson, 2003). This would be the case if chelation therapy was implemented using high doses of DFO to treat gross iron overload (Richardson, 2003). Clearly, this approach is not appropriate for patients with FA, in which iron loading is not as marked as in untreated β-thalassemia (Richardson, 2003). It is well known that DFO is a hydrophilic drug that does not penetrate mitochondrial membranes to bind intra-mitochondrial iron deposits (Richardson et al., 2001). The goal of an effective chelation regime for FA patients is to prevent mitochondrial iron accumulation using chelators that permeate the mitochondrion without causing marked body iron depletion and haematological toxicity (Richardson, 2003).

In this study, both PIH and DFO were used to limit iron accumulation as the phenotype is very severe in mutant mice, with death occurring at 10 weeks of age (Puccio et al., 2001). It is likely that such intense chelation therapy would not be required in human FA, as the progression is far slower (Pandolfo, 2003). Hence, only minimal chelation therapy with PIH alone *via* the oral route may be enough to prevent mitochondrial iron accumulation and its pathological effects.

Recently, a small clinical trial suggested the chelator deferiprone, may have favourable effects on preventing the neurological symptoms in FA (Boddaert et al., 2007). However, the role of iron chelation in producing this outcome was difficult to ascertain, as deferiprone was given at the same time as idebenone, which is known to ameliorate the neurological effects of FA (Di Prospero et al., 2007). Therefore, further studies with chelators alone in FA patients are essential.

In summary, there was a marked change in cardiac iron trafficking in MCK mutants and these studies show the mechanisms responsible for mitochondrial iron loading. Further, chelation therapy limits cardiac hypertrophy in the mutants, suggesting it may be beneficial for FA patients.

CHAPTER 5

CONDITIONAL FRATAXIN KNOCKOUT IN THE FRIEDREICH'S ATAXIA HEART: TREATMENT BY IRON SUPPLEMENTATION AND DEMONSTRATION OF THE CARDIAC CONTROL OF SYSTEMIC IRON METABOLISM

Whitnall M, Rahmanto YS, Guitérrez L, Lázaro FJ, Mikhael MR, Ponka P and Richardson DR (2011). Manuscript in preparation.

5.1 INTRODUCTION

Tissue iron loading can lead to toxicity, due to the ability of iron to redox cycle, producing cytotoxic radicals and inducing oxidative stress (Richardson, 2003). The potential of iron loading to become toxic may be more pronounced in the highly redox-active mitochondrial environment (Rötig et al., 1997). Mitochondrial iron loading has been associated with the pathogenesis of the severe autosomal recessive disease, FA (Richardson, 2003, Wong et al., 1999). This is supported by the location of iron accumulation at sites of neuronal and cardiac degeneration and the ability of iron chelation and anti-oxidant therapy alone, or in combination, to improve heart and/or neurological function in FA patients and animal models (Rustin et al., 1999, Velasco-Sanchez et al., 2010, Whitnall et al., 2008, Seznec et al., 2004).

While anti-oxidants and iron chelation alleviate symptoms of FA (Rustin et al., 1999, Velasco-Sanchez et al., 2010, Whitnall et al., 2008, Seznec et al., 2004), they do not address the genetic defect that underlies it (Seznec et al., 2004, Whitnall et al., 2008). Primarily, FA is caused by insufficient expression of the mitochondrial-associated protein, frataxin (Puccio et al., 2004, Rötig et al., 1997, Seznec et al., 2004), and the deleterious effect of mitochondrial iron loading is thought to act downstream of this (Whitnall et al., 2008, Puccio et al., 2001). While the precise molecular functions of frataxin remain unclear, converging evidence suggests its iron binding ability (Yoon and Cowan, 2003) facilitates a role as a mitochondrial iron chaperone for ISC generation (Wang and Craig, 2008, Leidgens et al., 2010, Richardson et al., 2010, Yoon and Cowan, 2003) and haem synthesis (Richardson et al., 2010, Yoon and Cowan, 2004, Lesuisse et al., 2003, Schoenfeld et al., 2005, Zhang et al., 2005b). Additionally, frataxin has also been linked to the detoxification of mitochondrial iron (O'Neill et al., 2005, Richardson et al., 2010). Similarly to FA, the deletion of frataxin *in vitro* and *in vivo* initiates a phenotype of ISC-deficiency and perturbed haem synthesis, with mitochondrial DNA damage, mitochondrial iron overload and oxidative stress, culminating in cardiac and neuronal degeneration (Huang et al., 2009, Puccio et al., 2001, Rötig et al., 1997, Wilson and Roof, 1997). Given the absolute necessity for ISC proteins in vital processes such as respiration (*e.g.,* SDHA) and haem synthesis (*e.g.,* ferrochelatase; Fech) (Napier et al., 2005), therapies that are unable to correct this ISC deficiency will only offer a partial rescue of the pathology observed in FA. Currently, no effective strategies exist that address the reconstitution of iron into the mitochondrial iron requiring pathways of ISC and haem synthesis.

Recent *in vitro* and *in vivo* studies have demonstrated that in addition to mitochondrial iron-loading, down-regulation of frataxin also causes cytosolic iron deficiency (Li et al., 2008, Whitnall et al., 2008, Huang et al., 2009). Indeed, my studies in Chapter 4 demonstrated that within the cardiomyocyte, deletion of frataxin increases iron uptake *via* up-regulation of TfR1, with subsequent targeting of iron to the mitochondrion causing mitochondrial iron overload (Whitnall et al., 2008). In contrast, the proportion of cytosolic iron and expression of the cytosolic storage protein, H-ferritin, decreases after frataxin deletion, indicating the cytosol is iron deficient (Whitnall et al., 2008). These studies dissected the intracellular and molecular disruptions to iron trafficking pathways that arise from frataxin deficiency. Further understanding of FA pathogenesis will provide further clues regarding the function of frataxin and the extent of its involvement in mitochondrial, intracellular and potentially systemic iron metabolism.

Cardiomyopathy is a frequent cause of death in FA (Delatycki et al., 2000). While mitochondrial-iron loading appears to be important in the pathogenesis of this disease, cytosolic iron-deficiency could also play a role in the pathogenesis of FA. Indeed, iron deficiency induces cell cycle arrest and leads to apoptosis and cell death (Yu et al., 2007). Considering this, we examined the therapeutic effect of dietary iron supplementation on reconstituting ISC deficient enzymes and correcting the cytosolic iron-deficiency. These studies were performed using the MCK frataxin mutant mouse, which, as outlined in Section 4.2.1, lack frataxin in the mutant heart and skeletal muscle only (Puccio et al., 2001). Mutants exhibit classical traits of the cardiomyopathy characteristic of FA, including cardiac hypertrophy, ISC enzyme deficiency and mitochondrial iron accumulation (Puccio et al., 2001, Whitnall et al., 2008, Sutak et al., 2008, Huang et al., 2009). The data presented herein demonstrate that iron supplementation limits cardiac hypertrophy. It also reveals a novel effect of frataxin deletion on systemic iron metabolism, whereby frataxin deletion and consequential induction of cytosolic iron deficiency in the heart, induces a signaling mechanism to increase systemic iron uptake that is probably aimed at restoring cardiac iron balance. Finally, to obtain more information regarding the form of iron accumulating in mutant mitochondria, size exclusion chromatography, transmission electron microscopy and magnetic measurements were performed. These studies demonstrate, that iron accumulating in mutant mitochondria has characteristics of well crystallised, anti-ferromagnetic mineral iron aggregates distinctly different to ferritin.

5.2 MATERIALS AND METHODS

5.2.1 Animals and Genotyping

MCK mutant and WT mice were used (Section 4.2.1), and genotyping performed on isolated genomic tail DNA as in Section 4.2.2.

5.2.2 Dietary Iron Supplementation Studies

Mice were fed a normal iron diet (0.02% iron/kg) or high iron diet (2.00% iron/kg) (Specialty Feeds, Perth, Western Australia) from 4.5 to 8.5 weeks of age. After this time, mice were sacrificed and organ weights assessed (Section 2.2.2). Harvested tissues were used for histochemistry (as per Section 2.3.3), measurement of tissue iron stores (as per Section 2.3.2), IRP-RNA binding activity assays (as per Section 2.6) and western analysis as below.

5.2.3 Western Analysis

Protein was isolated from heart and liver tissue as described in Section 2.5.1. Western blot analysis was performed as per Section 2.5.2, using antibodies against ferroportin1, frataxin, GAPDH, H-ferritin, SDHA and TfR1 at dilutions listed in section 4.2.5. Additionally, ferrochelatase (Fech; Prof. Harry Dailey, University of Georgia, Biomedical and Health Sciences Institute, USA) was used at a dilution of 1:2000, haem oxygenase (Hmox1) at 1:500 (Stressgen, Plymouth Meeting, USA), hemojuvelin (Hjv) at 1:2000 (Prof. Seppo Parkkila, University of Tampere, Institute of Medical Technology, Tampere, Finland) and IRP2 at 1:500 (Novus Biologicals,

Littleton, USA). Densitometric analysis was performed as per Section 2.8.1.

5.2.4 Size-Exclusion Chromatography

MCK mutant and WT mice were i.v. injected with ^{59}Fe-Tf as per Section 2.7. Mice were sacrificed 24 h post i.v. injection of ^{59}Fe-Tf, the hearts removed and washed, and cytosolic and mitochondrial fractions prepared as per Section 2.7. Mitochondrial fractions were sonicated on ice in lysis buffer (10 mM HEPES, 140 mM NaCl, 1.5% triton X-100, pH 8.0, supplemented with complete protease inhibitor$^{®}$) and centrifuged at min 16,500 g/45 min/4 $^{\circ}$C and the soluble mitochondrial fraction (supernatant) collected.

Cytosolic and stromal mitochondrial membrane (SMM) fractions were incubated for 2 h at 4 $^{\circ}$C in the presence or absence of 2 mM DFO (Novartis). Size-exclusion chromatography was performed using a Superdex 200 HR 10/30 column (Amersham Biosciences) and protein fractions eluted with 20 mM HEPES and 140 mM NaCl (pH 8.0; flow rate 0.5 mL/min) using a BioLogic Fast Pressure Liquid Chromatography System (BioRad). The ^{59}Fe in eluted fractions was measured using a Wallac WIZARD 1480 γ-counter (PerkinElmer). Between samples, the column was extensively washed with DFO (2 mM) and deionised water to elute ^{59}Fe and proteins that may have become trapped on the column. This avoided cross-contamination between different samples.

5.2.5 Transmission Electron Microscopy

MCK mutant and WT mice were anaesthetised with isofluorane (Abbott Australasia Pty Ltd). To flush blood from the system, an incision was made in the right atrium and warmed fixative solution (2% paraformaldehyde and 2% glutaraldehyde in 0.1 M phosphate buffer, pH 7.2) injected into the left ventricle. Heart and liver tissues were harvested and fixed whole for 1 h/4 °C before careful dissection into 1 mm^3 pieces and further fixation overnight at 4 °C. Samples were then washed three times with 0.4 M HEPES (pH 7.2) and post-fixed with 1% osmium tetroxide (Sigma-Aldrich) for   30 min/4 °C. Samples were again washed three times in HEPES, and then dehydrated in graded ethanol solutions (30, 50, 70, 90, 100%) for 10 min each at 4 °C. Infiltration was performed gradually through LR White resin (LRW; Sigma-Aldrich) : ethanol solutions (1:3, 1:1, 3:1) for 30 min each at 4 °C, LRW (100%) overnight at 4 °C and three changes of LRW (100%) for 12 h each at 4 °C. Samples were embedded in LRW and polymerised at 60 °C for 48 h. Ultra-thin sections (40-60 nm) were collected on Formvar-coated gold grids (Electron Microscopy Sciences, Hatfield, USA). Micrographs were taken by Dr Lucia Guitérrez (Instituto de Ciencia de Materiales de Madrid, Spain) on a Philips Tecnai 20 transmission electron microscope (Amsterdam, Netherlands) operated at 200 kV equipped with an energy dispersive X-ray spectrometer (Philips). This allowed us to confirm the presence of within the field of view.

5.2.6 Magnetic Susceptibility Measurements

Heart samples were freeze-dried in a Heto PowerDry PL3000 Freeze Dryer (Thermo Fisher Scientific), ground to powder to ensure homogeneity and placed in gelatine capsules ready for measurement. Magnetic susceptibility measurements were determined by Prof. Francisco Lázaro (Departamento de Ciencia y Tecnología de Materiales y Fluidos, Spain) using an MPMS-

XL magnetometer (Quantum Design, San Diego, USA) equipped with an alternating current (AC) susceptibility option. Measurements were performed at an exciting AC field of 0.4 milliTesla and frequency of 10 Hz in the temperature range of 1.8 – 300 K. Following magnetic characterisation, tissues were analysed *via* ICP-AES (Section 2.6) to ensure magnetism of the sample could be ascribed to the presence of iron and to calculate the magnetic effective moment (Lázaro et al., 2007). Diamagnetic contributions which originate from the metallic sample holder were taken into account and corrected for.

5.3 RESULTS

5.3.1 Iron Supplementation Delays Weight Loss and Limits Cardiac Hypertrophy

Studies in Chapter 4 demonstrated that the MCK mutant heart is in a state of cytosolic iron-deficiency (Whitnall et al., 2008), and deficiency of ISCs has been noted to precede cardiomyopathy in these animals (Seznec et al., 2004). Considering this, the therapeutic contribution of dietary iron supplementation in the restoration of these deficiencies was examined. Such a treatment strategy may lead to the re-constitution of iron in ISC enzymes such as complex II of the respiratory chain, *i.e.,* SDHA, which is deficient in the MCK mutant mouse (Puccio et al., 2001, Sutak et al., 2008).

In these experiments, WT and mutant mice were maintained on a diet of normal iron (0.02% iron/kg) or high iron (2.00% iron/kg) from 4.5 weeks of age, until the conclusion of the study when mice were 8.5 weeks of age. Such a protocol has been shown previously to lead to iron-loading in mice

(Sekyere et al., 2006). The starting age of 4.5 weeks was used as at this age, mutant mice do not demonstrate any overt phenotypic changes, as described earlier (Section 4.3.1) (Puccio et al., 2001, Whitnall et al., 2008).

5.3.1.1 Animal Growth After Iron Supplementation

No significant differences were observed in the growth of WT mice fed either diet (Figure 5.1A). As previously shown (Section 4.3.4.2) (Whitnall et al., 2008), mutant mice begin to lose weight between 6-7 weeks of age. Interestingly, in high iron diet fed mutants, weight loss was less marked than normal iron diet fed mutants from 7.5 weeks of age (Figure 5.1A). At the conclusion of the study, there was a slight (but not significant) increase in the body weight of high- compared to normal-iron diet fed mutants.

5.3.1.2 Cardiac Hypertrophy After Iron Supplementation

Heart weight and the heart-to-body weight ratio can be used as a measure of cardiac hypertrophy (Puccio et al., 2001, Whitnall et al., 2008). Consistent with previous studies (Puccio et al., 2001, Whitnall et al., 2008), normal iron diet fed mutants showed a significant increase ($p < 0.001$) in the heart-to-body weight ratio compared to their normal iron diet fed WT counterparts (Figure 5.1B). Mutants receiving the high iron diet also experienced a significant increase ($p < 0.001$) in the heart to body weight ratio compared to their high iron fed diet WT counterparts. However, the extent of cardiac enlargement was significantly less ($p < 0.001$) in high iron diet fed mutants compared to when these mutants were fed a normal iron diet (Figure 5.1B). Collectively, these data indicate that dietary iron supplementation moderates, but does not totally rescue the cardiac hypertrophy of the mutant mouse probably because the extra iron does not totally replace frataxin function which is needed for ISC synthesis *etc*.

5.3.1.3 Organ Iron Content After Iron Supplementation

To demonstrate the effect of dietary iron loading on organ iron levels, heart, liver, spleen and kidney were dissected, extensively washed and their iron levels directly measured using ICP-AES (Figures 5.1C-F). Cardiac iron levels were significantly ($p < 0.001$) higher in both normal- and high-iron diet fed mutants compared to their WT counterparts (Figure 5.1C). As shown in Chapter 4 and in previous studies (Puccio et al., 2001, Whitnall et al., 2008), this is due to iron accumulation in the mitochondrial compartment. Furthermore, there was a slight, yet significant ($p < 0.05$), increase in the cardiac iron levels of mutants fed a high iron diet (490.6 $\pm$ 11.4 μg/g; $n = 27$) compared to a normal iron diet (460.0 $\pm$ 13.7 μg/g; $n = 24$; Figure 5.1C).

Concentrations of iron in the liver, spleen and kidney (Figures 5.1D-F), were significantly greater in high iron diet fed WT and mutant mice compared to their normal iron diet fed counterparts. This result is consistent with previous findings in murine studies (Ward et al., 2003), and demonstrates the iron enriched diet was successful in iron loading the mice. The largest increase in iron levels in high iron diet fed mice was observed in the liver, consistent with the known role of this organ in iron storage (Drysdale and Munro, 1966, Harrison and Arosio, 1996, Trinder et al., 1996). Of particular interest were the significant increases ($p < 0.001$) in iron levels found in the liver, spleen and kidney of mutant relative to WT mice fed the normal diet (Figures 5.1D-F). This indicates that deletion of frataxin in the heart and skeletal muscle leads to a systemic alteration of iron metabolism, as described in our earlier studies (Huang et al., 2009).

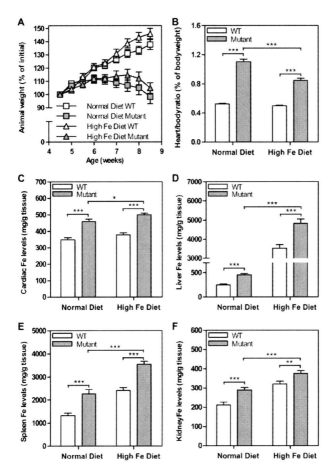

Figure 5.1 Dietary iron supplementation does (A) not significantly rescue weight loss in mutant mice, but (B) limits cardiac hypertrophy. Frataxin-deficiency in the mutant heart leads to iron loading in the (C) heart, and (D) systemic iron loading in the liver, (E) spleen and (F) kidney. WT and mutant mice were fed a normal (0.02% iron/kg) or high (2.00% iron/kg) iron diet from 4.5 to 8.5 weeks of age. **(A)** During this time, mice were weighed twice-weekly until the conclusion of the study. Upon sacrifice, the heart was washed, weighed and **(B)** heart to body weight ratios calculated as an assessment of cardiac hypertrophy. **(C-F)** Total iron concentration was assessed in the washed heart, liver, spleen and kidney in mice from **(A and B)**, using ICP-AES. Results in **(A and B)** are mean $\pm$ SEM (n = 30 – 38 mice) and **(C-F)** are mean $\pm$ SEM (n = 24 - 30 mice). $* p < 0.05; ** p < 0.01; *** p < 0.001$.

5.3.2 Effect of Iron Supplementation on Expression of Proteins in the Heart and Liver

Western analysis was performed to examine the effect of dietary iron supplementation on the expression of proteins involved in the metabolism and regulation of iron in the heart and liver to further examine the surprising systemic effect of frataxin deletion in the heart and skeletal muscle.

5.3.2.1 Frataxin Deficiency Does Not Lead to the Normal Physiologic Response to Dietary Iron Loading in the Mutant Heart

First, it is important to note that while there was a marked and significant ($p < 0.001$) decrease in frataxin expression in the mutant heart, frataxin was not entirely ablated. Very slight levels of frataxin were detected in the mutant (Figure 5.2A). As noted in Chapter 4 (Section 4.3.1) (Whitnall et al., 2008), this is due to other cells within the total heart homogenate apart from cardiomyocytes *e.g.,* fibroblasts, which are not targeted by the conditional knockout strategy. The high iron diet relative to the normal diet did not significantly alter frataxin expression in either the mutant or WT mice (Figure 5.2A).

As demonstrated in Chapter 4, frataxin deficiency in the mutant heart markedly alters cardiac iron metabolism (Huang et al., 2009, Whitnall et al., 2008). Indeed, similarly to the results in Chapter 4 (Huang et al., 2009, Whitnall et al., 2008) using mutant relative to WT mice fed a normal diet, there was up-regulation of TfR1 and down-regulation of H-ferritin and ferroportin1, accompanied by increased IRP2 expression (Figure 5.2A) and RNA-binding activity (Figure 5.3). It is well known that the TfR1 is crucial for   Tf-bound iron uptake, which is the main pathway of cellular iron internalisation under physiological conditions (Hentze and Kuhn, 1996, Richardson and Ponka, 1997). Typically, and as expected from IRP-IRE theory in cells loaded with iron (Richardson and Ponka, 1997), following feeding of a high iron diet, a significant ($p < 0.01$) decrease in TfR1 expression was observed in the hearts of WT mice fed a high- compared to normal-iron diet (Figure 5.2A). In clear contrast, TfR1 expression was not significantly altered in hearts of mutants fed a high- relative to normal-iron diet (Figure 5.2A). This indicated that in the mutant, frataxin deficiency does not lead to the normal protective response mediated by the IRP-IRE mechanism (Hentze and Kuhn, 1996) to down-regulate TfR1 in response to increased cellular iron levels.

A significant increase ($p < 0.05$) in expression of the cytosolic iron storage protein,   H-ferritin, was observed in WT mice fed a high- compared to normal-iron diet   (Figure 5.2A). This is consistent with the well known response of ferritin to sequester increased amounts of iron entering cells following iron loading (Figure 5.1C). However, in the hearts of mutants fed a high iron diet, H-ferritin, remained significantly down-regulated in comparison to WT mice on either diet. Again, this indicates that frataxin deficiency did not lead to the normal regulation of iron metabolism in the hearts of mutants fed a high iron diet fed. Surprisingly, ferroportin1 expression did not significantly change in the hearts of WT mice fed the normal compared to high iron diet. IRP2 protein expression was virtually undetectable in WT animals fed a normal diet as well as in their counterparts fed a high iron diet (Figure 5.2A). In contrast, as shown previously, in mutants fed a normal diet, there was pronounced IRP2 expression, but this was not reduced in mutants fed a high iron diet. Clearly, this latter observation in mutants is in direct contrast to IRP-IRE theory, where increased cellular iron levels leads to reduced IRP2 protein levels (Hentze et al., 2010). Collectively, for the first time, these observations above examining the protein expression of TfR1, ferritin and IRP2, indicate that deletion of frataxin prevents the normal regulation of intracellular iron metabolism in response to altered iron levels.

In addition to the proteins involved in iron metabolism that are post-transcriptionally controlled by IRP2 above (*i.e.*, TfR1, H-ferritin and ferroportin1), results in Chapter 4 (Figures 4.1 and 4.4) (Whitnall et al., 2008) and in our previous studies (Huang et al., 2009), and the current investigation (Figure 5.2A), demonstrated that Fech, MIT ferritin, hemojuvelin (Hjv) and SDHA expression were decreased in mutants relative to WT mice fed a normal diet. Feeding mutant mice an iron-loaded diet, did not alter expression of these molecules relative to mice fed a normal diet (Figure 5.2A). Furthermore, as we have also shown previously (Huang et al., 2009), in this investigation (Figure 5.2A) haem oxygenase 1 (Hmox1) was increased in mutants relative to WT mice fed a normal diet. However, the iron-loaded diet did not alter this expression pattern. These studies demonstrated that the expression of these proteins in the mutants could not be altered through iron supplementation.

A - Heart

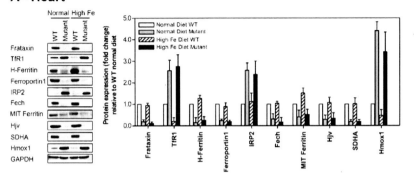

B - Liver

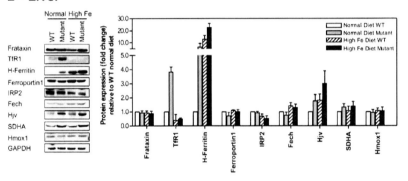

Figure 5.2 Frataxin deficiency in the heart prevents the normal physiological response to dietary iron loading in the mutant heart and causes systemic alterations to iron metabolism related proteins in the mutant liver. Tissue was collected from mice in Figure 5.1 and western blot and densitometric analysis performed examining iron metabolism related proteins in normal- and high- iron diet fed WT and mutant **(A)** hearts and **(B)** livers. Western panels are typical experiments, and densitometry is mean ± SD (3-5 experiments).

5.3.2.2 RNA-Binding Activity of IRP2 is not Decreased in Mutants Hearts by Iron Loading

In vivo, intracellular iron metabolism is regulated by IRP2, which influences the expression of its target genes that contain an iron-responsive element (IRE), including TfR1, ferritin, ferroportin1 *e.t.c.* (Li et al., 2008, Meyron-Holtz et al., 2004b, Meyron-Holtz et al., 2004a). In contrast, IRP1 is thought to play less of a role *in vivo* in regulating the metabolism of iron (Meyron-Holtz et al., 2004a, Meyron-Holtz et al., 2004b). As demonstrated in Chapter 4 (Section 4.3.2) (Whitnall et al., 2008), in the current investigation (Figures 5.3A and B), IRP2-RNA binding activity was significantly increased ($p < 0.01$) in mutants relative to WT mice fed a normal diet, and this is probably responsible for the up-regulation of TfR1 and down-regulation of both H-ferritin and ferroportin1 expression in mutant mice (Figure 5.2A). In contrast, IRP1-RNA binding activity did not alter between the mutant and WT animals either in the presence or absence of β-ME (Figures 5.3A and B) which converts IRP1 from its non-RNA binding cytosolic aconitase form to its RNA-binding protein (Meyron-Holtz et al., 2004a). This supports previous investigations by others that demonstrated IRP1 is insensitive to cellular iron status *in vivo* (Meyron-Holtz et al., 2004a, Meyron-Holtz et al., 2004b) and supports the role of IRP2 as the primary regulator of iron homeostasis *in vivo* (Meyron-Holtz et al., 2004b, Whitnall et al., 2008), at least in the heart.

Of interest, the high IRP2-RNA binding activity observed in mutants fed a normal diet was not significantly affected when these animals were fed a high iron diet (Figures 5.3A and B). This finding agrees with our western blotting studies examining IRP2 protein levels (Figure 5.2A), and occurs despite a significant ($p < 0.05$) increase in cardiac iron levels in mutants fed a high- relative to normal-iron diet (Figure 5.1C). Considering that IRP2 responds to changes in cytosolic iron levels (Rouault, 2009), these results indicate that dietary iron supplementation of the mutants did not lead to IRP2 down-regulation. As such, the high iron diet did not offset the cytosolic iron-deficiency present in the MCK mutant heart.

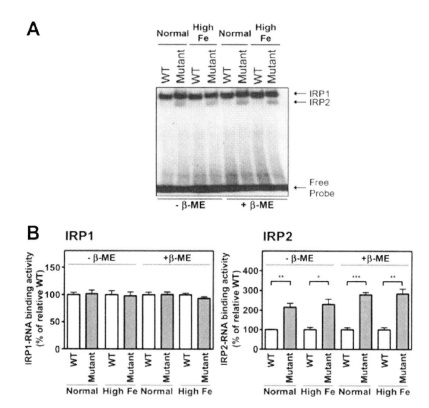

Figure 5.3 IRP2-RNA binding activity in the heart is increased in mutant mice relative to their WT counterparts fed a normal iron diet and is not affected by a high iron diet. (A) IRP-RNA binding activity was assayed by gel-retardation analysis. WT and mutant mice were treated as in Figure 5.1. Upon sacrifice, the heart was washed and homogenized in Munro buffer. Equal amounts of heart extract were assayed in the absence and presence of β-mercaptoethanol (β-ME). Results in (A) are from a typical experiment, whereas the densitometry in (B) is mean $\pm$ SD of 3-4 experiments. * $p < 0.05$; ** $p < 0.01$; *** $p < 0.001$.

5.3.2.3 Systemic Effects in the Liver Following Frataxin Deletion in the Heart and Skeletal Muscle

As shown in Figures 5.1D-F, there was a significant increase in the level of iron in the liver, spleen and kidney of normal iron diet fed mutants relative to their WT counterparts. This observation implies that ablation of frataxin in the heart not only alters cardiac iron metabolism, but also affects systemic iron metabolism. Considering the liver is a central regulator of systemic iron metabolism (Hentze et al., 2010), we examined the expression of iron-related proteins in this organ, in which frataxin expression is unaltered (Figure 5.2B). Moreover, we compared the expression of these proteins in the liver after WT and mutant mice were fed a normal and high iron diet, to the effects observed in the heart (Figure 5.2A).

The MCK conditional frataxin knockout mouse model leads to the deletion of frataxin in the heart and skeletal muscle, but not in other organs (Puccio et al., 2001, Huang et al., 2009). In the liver, no changes in frataxin expression were observed comparing WT and mutant mice fed either the normal- or high-iron diet (Figure 5.2B). This indicates that the significant ($p < 0.001$) increase in liver iron loading in high iron diet fed mice (Figure 5.1D), does not significantly affect frataxin expression.

As found in the hearts of mutant mice fed a normal diet (Figure 5.1A), TfR1 expression in the liver was also was significantly up-regulated ($p < 0.001$; Figure 5.2B) in normal iron diet fed mutants compared to their WT counterparts. However, in contrast to the heart (Figure 5.1A), TfR1 expression in the liver of high iron diet fed mutants was markedly and significantly ($p < 0.001$) down-regulated. This observation demonstrated that unlike the heart, the physiological response to iron loading in the liver was intact. Examining WT mice, a significant ($p < 0.05$) decrease in TfR1 expression in the liver was found comparing normal iron diet fed WTs to high iron diet fed WTs (Figure 5.2B). While the changes observed in the livers of high iron diet fed WT mice are consistent with previous well documented findings following dietary iron loading (Robb and Wessling-Resnick, 2004), the reason for the increase in TfR1 in normal iron diet fed mutants is unclear, especially considering the significantly ($p < 0.001$) higher liver iron levels in the mutant (Figure 5.1D). However, these changes can probably be explained by the deletion of frataxin in the heart. Indeed, the marked iron loading in the liver, spleen and kidney of normal iron diet fed mutants, could be part of a compensatory systemic alteration that increases iron levels in an attempt to overcome the cytosolic iron deficiency in the heart.

In direct contrast to the results in the hearts of normal iron diet fed mice (Figure 5.2A), in the liver, H-ferritin expression was significantly ($p < 0.001$) greater in normal iron diet fed mutants compared with their WT counterparts (Figure 5.2B). This finding reflects the significantly ($p < 0.001$) higher liver iron levels in the normal iron diet fed mutant (Figure 5.1D). The extent of H-ferritin expression was greater in WT and mutant mice fed a high iron diet relative to those fed a normal diet, in accordance with the physiological function of the liver as a major site for iron storage (Drysdale and Munro, 1966, Harrison and Arosio, 1996, Trinder et al., 1996).

The expression of ferroportin1 and Hmox1 were not markedly altered in WT and mutant mice fed a normal diet or an iron loaded diet (Figure 5.2B). A slight but significant ($p < 0.05$) increase in liver ferrochelatase expression was observed in both high- compared to normal-iron diet fed WTs and high- compared to normal-iron diet fed mutants (Figure 5.2B). Interestingly, Hjv expression in the liver (Figure 5.2B) in response to iron-loading was opposite to the response that was observed in the heart (Figure 5.2A). In fact, mutants demonstrated significantly higher Hjv expression than their WT counterparts when fed either a normal- or high-iron loaded diet ($p < 0.001$ in normal iron diet fed mutants compared with their WT counterparts, and $p < 0.05$ in high iron diet fed mutants compared with their WT counterparts).

Again, in contrast to the results obtained in the heart (Figure 5.2A), there was no significant difference in IRP2 protein expression in the liver between WT and mutant mice fed a normal diet, despite the significantly ($p < 0.001$) greater iron levels in the liver of the mutant (Figure 5.1D). However, relative to the normal iron diet, for both WT and mutant mice, the high iron diet led to a significant decrease in IRP2 expression, in agreement with the iron-mediated degradation of IRP2 (Rouault, 2006).

Another unexpected finding in the liver of the mutant was that SDHA expression was significantly ($p < 0.05$) greater than that observed for the WT mice fed either a normal- or high-iron diet (Figure 5.2B). The reason for this alteration remains unknown, but could represent an attempt at the systemic level to compensate for the metabolic defect in the heart and skeletal muscle induced by frataxin deficiency. Our previous studies have shown that a variety of molecular mechanisms within the mutant heart are induced in an attempt to ameliorate the deficiency in energy metabolism (Sutak et al., 2008). Considering the alterations in iron metabolism at a systemic level reported for the liver above, other metabolic alterations that act to aid the vital functioning of the failing heart in the MCK mutant, could also be expected.

The results above indicate that frataxin deletion in the heart and skeletal muscle leads to marked alterations in the regulation of iron metabolism in the liver. Indeed, the alterations in expression of many molecules involved in iron processing in the mutant appear to occur in an attempt to increase both iron uptake (TfR1) and storage (ferritin). The loading of iron not only in the mutant liver, but in the spleen and kidney, likewise supports this hypothesis. This may represent a compensatory systemic response to aid the cytosolic iron deficiency observed in the heart, demonstrating the heart's essential requirement for iron, and crucial role in whole body functioning.

5.3.3 Iron Accumulates in the Mutant Heart in a Unique Form

While the occurrence of iron accumulation in the heart of FA patients (Richardson, 2003) and the MCK mutant mouse (Puccio et al., 2001, Whitnall et al., 2008) is well documented, little is known about the exact molecular form of these iron deposits. This is important for understanding the metabolic defect at a mechanistic level, but also in terms of aiding the development of new therapeutics to treat FA. To this extent, the techniques of size-exclusion chromatography, transmission electron microscopy (TEM) and alternating current (AC) magnetic susceptibility were used to try and elucidate the form and characteristics of iron that accumulates in the frataxin-deficient mutant heart.

5.3.3.1 Marked Alterations Exist in ^{59}Fe Distribution in the Mutant Heart

To understand how cardiac iron is distributed within subcellular compartments, 9-week-old WT and mutant mice were radio-labelled *via* tail vein injection using ^{59}Fe-Tf and then sacrificed 96 h later. Lysates derived from cytosolic and SMM fractions were then incubated in the presence or absence of DFO (2 mM) and separated based on molecular weight *via* size-exclusion chromatography using fast pressure liquid chromatography. DFO was added to bind low M_r inorganic iron that could be present in fractions, and is known to become bound to the size exclusion media used for chromatographic separation (Richardson et al., 1996).

Eluted fractions were analysed for their content of ^{59}Fe using a γ-scintillation counter. Cytosolic fractions from WT and mutant mice demonstrated 1 major ^{59}Fe containing peak at fraction 15 and two substantially smaller peaks in fractions 20-22 and fraction 24 (Figure 5.4A). The addition of DFO had no marked effect on this elution pattern with no significant difference being observed over three experiments for most of the observed peaks. However, upon addition of DFO to mutant cytosolic lysates, a minor extra peak was identified at fractions 27-28 that was not observed upon the addition of DFO to the WT cytosol (Figure 5.4A).

Differences were observed in the proportion of cytosolic ^{59}Fe within these peaks between the WT and mutant mice, in particular, incorporation of ^{59}Fe in fraction 15, which was markedly greater in the WT than the mutant (Figure 5.4A). Studies demonstrated that purified ferritin co-eluted at fraction 15 (data not shown), suggesting that this peak corresponded to ferritin, which is consistent with its function as the major iron-storage protein in the cell (Arosio et al., 2009). These results agree with our previous studies demonstrating that ferritin is markedly decreased in the mutant relative to the WT mice (Whitnall et al., 2008, Huang et al., 2009). Furthermore, ^{59}Fe in the total cytosolic compartment was greater in WT (89,789 CPM) compared with mutant mice (48,296 CPM), confirming the mutant cytosol was in an iron deficient state, as previously demonstrated (Chapter 4) (Whitnall et al., 2008).

The elution of ^{59}Fe from the SMM fraction (Figure 5.4B) was distinctly different to that obtained for the cytosolic fraction (Figure 5.4A). WT and mutant lysates from the SMM fraction produced ^{59}Fe peaks in fractions 11-13, 15, 20 and 27-28 (Figure 5.4B). But again, differences were observed in the proportion of ^{59}Fe incorporated in each fraction comparing WT with mutant mice (Figure 5.4B). Mutant mice are known to have markedly increased concentrations of iron within the mitochondrial compartment (Puccio et al., 2001, Whitnall et al., 2008). Interestingly, only after incubation of the lysates with DFO was sufficient ^{59}Fe eluted from the column to reflect this. In the absence of DFO, only 58% of the ^{59}Fe that was loaded onto the column was eluted from the mutant mitochondrial lysate, compared to 74% after incubation with DFO. Indeed, addition of DFO induced a pronounced and significant increase in the elution of ^{59}Fe that was derived from lysates of mutant mice in fraction 27-28 relative to the lysates from WT animals treated in the same way (Figure 5.4*B*). Fractions 27-28 correlate to those observed after a solution of the DFO-^{59}Fe complex was passed through the column alone. Hence, it was evident that the majority of ^{59}Fe in the mutant mitochondrion became adsorbed with high affinity to the column. Notably, a similar adsorption of ^{59}Fe to size exclusion chromatography media with its subsequent liberation by DFO has been observed previously in studies examining mitochondrial ^{59}Fe accumulation in reticulocytes treated with the heme synthesis inhibitor, succinylacetone (Richardson et al., 1996).

Collectively, these results demonstrate that marked differences exist in the distribution of iron in the cytosol and SMM fractions of mutant compared with WT mice. Furthermore, these experiments also indicated that the iron accumulation within the mutant mitochondrion is marked and can be solubilised by DFO after becoming adsorbed to size-exclusion chromatography media.

A - Cytosol

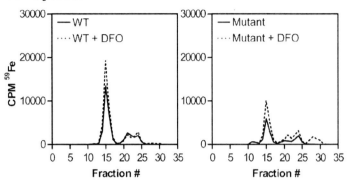

B - Mitochondria

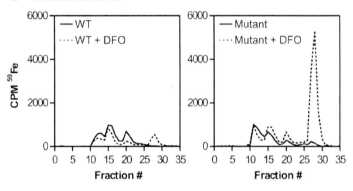

Figure 5.4 Size-exclusion chromatography of cytosolic and stromal mitochondrial membrane fractions demonstrates marked alterations exist in ^{59}Fe distribution in the mutant heart relative to its wild-type counterpart. Total ^{59}Fe in the mutant mitochondrion is only recovered following treatment of the lysate with the iron chelator, desferrioxamine (DFO). WT and mutant mice were injected i.v. *via* the tail vein with ^{59}Fe-Tf (0.6 mg) and sacrificed after 96 h. The hearts were thoroughly washed, homogenised at 4 ^{o}C and **(A)** cytosolic and **(B)** stromal mitochondrial membrane fractions prepared for size-exclusion chromatography by centrifugation at 16,500 g/45 min/4 ^{o}C. Fractions were incubated at 4 ^{o}C for 2 h in the presence or absence of DFO (2 mM) and loaded onto a Superdex 200 HR 10/30 column. ^{59}Fe was measured using a γ-counter and counts recovered following elution of the lysate were calculated. Results are a typical experiment from 3 performed.

5.3.3.2 Transmission Electron Microscopy Demonstrates Ferritin Iron Accumulation in the Mutant Liver and Non Ferritin Iron Accumulation in the Mutant Heart

To characterise the form of iron accumulating in the mutant heart, unstained tissue sections were examined using TEM (Figures 5.5A and B). Unstained sections were specifically used in the current study, as staining with uranyl acetate and lead citrate in conventional TEM, can introduce heavy metal clusters that can be confused with endogenous iron containing molecules such as ferritin. In all studies, the presence of iron was confirmed by energy-dispersive spectrometry (data not shown).

Figures 5.5A and B show micrographs of unstained liver and heart sections, respectively, from mutant mice only. While WT sections were also examined, no iron particles could be observed in the WT heart (data not shown). In the WT liver, particles of iron were similar to those in the mutant liver (Figure 5.5Ai and ii), but appeared at a much lower frequency (data not shown). For these reasons, only sections from the mutant heart and liver, in which large concentrations of iron are present (Figures 5.1C and D) and visible (Figures 5.5A and B), were included herein.

Clear differences were observed between the form of iron accumulating in the mutant liver (Figure 5.5A) compared to the mutant heart (Figure 5.5B). In the liver of mutant mice, at low magnification (Figure 5.5Ai), iron appears in isolated, electron-dense particles. Upon examination of the structure of these particles at higher magnification (Figure 5.5Aii inset), they appear to be composed of an electron-dense core surrounded by an electron lucent shell with a diameter of approximately 5-8 nm (Figure 5.5Aii inset). This observation is consistent with the TEM structure of cytosolic ferritin (Iancu, 1992), in which the electron lucent protein shell, evident upon staining with uranyl acetate, prevents mutual contact of the particles (Quintana, 2007). In contrast, ferritin particles were not evident in the mutant heart (Figure 5.5B), despite significant iron-loading of this tissue (Figure 5.1C). Unlike the mutant liver, iron in the mutant heart seen at low power, is in large heterogeneous aggregates, which measure 100-400 nm in diameter. These aggregates most likely have a mitochondrial location, given the elliptical shape of the discreet boundary, that is probably the mitochondrial membrane, surrounding them (see arrow in Figure 5.5Bi). At higher magnification (Figure 5.5Bii), the aggregate was observed to be composed of much smaller, irregularly shaped, electron-dense particles (Figure 5.5Bii inset) which ranged from 1-14 nm in diameter. Unlike the ferritin molecules in the liver that were observed at the same magnification (Figure 5.5Aii), contact is obvious between the iron particles, suggesting they lack a protein shell.

5.3.3.3 Magnetic Susceptibility Measurements Demonstrate Anti-ferromagnetic Iron in the Mutant Heart is Not Present in Ferritin

Under normal physiological conditions, biological tissues possess magnetic properties that are largely due to the presence and form of iron within the tissue (Lázaro et al., 2007). Hence, these magnetic properties can provide information regarding the state of the iron present. Given this, we performed magnetic AC susceptibility measurements to further characterise the form of iron accumulating in the mutant heart. Tissue from 4- and 9-week-old mice was used, since 4 week-old mutants demonstrate no detectable mitochondrial iron accumulation, and therefore provide an appropriate negative control to the 9 week-old mutants where mitochondrial iron deposits are marked and the cardiac pathology is obvious (Puccio et al., 2001, Whitnall et al., 2008). Clearly, the 4- and

9-week-old WT mice have no mitochondrial iron-loading and are appropriate controls to the mutants at each of these ages.

Figure 5.5*C* demonstrates the in-phase component of the AC magnetic susceptibility of cardiac tissue from 4- and 9-week-old WT and mutant mice, which is an indicator of biomineralisation and the spin of electrons within cardiac tissue (Lazaro et al., 2005, Lázaro et al., 2007). Notably, the AC susceptibility from 9 week old mutants is distinctly different to that of the 4 week-old mutants and the 4- and 9- week-old WT mice, indicating a difference in the form of iron present. The structural organisation of iron ions within the sample can be assessed by calculating the magnetic effective moment (μ_{eff}) per iron ion in the tissue (Lazaro et al., 2005, Lázaro et al., 2007). At   4 weeks of age, no significant difference exists between the μ_{eff} of WT (2.87 ± 0.22 μ_B) and mutant (2.70 ± 0.21 μ_B) mice. However at 9 weeks of age, the μ_{eff} becomes significantly ($p < 0.05$) lower in mutant (2.17 ± 0.02 μ_B) compared to WT mice   (2.64 ± 0.16 μ_B).

Candidate species of iron that could account for the change in AC magnetic susceptibility and reduction in μ_{eff} in 9 week-old mutants are: (i) a well crystallised, anti-ferromagnetic mineral iron aggregate (*i.e.,* an iron compound with anti-parallel spin alignment of electrons); or (ii) an ISC-containing molecule, whose μ_{eff} decreases from 3.24 μ_B to 0.38 μ_B with addition of iron atoms within the molecule (Li et al., 1996). However, the probability that an ISC is responsible for the reduction in μ_{eff} is unlikely, given that formation of ISCs is depressed in the absence of frataxin (Richardson et al., 2010, Huang et al., 2009). In agreement with our molecular investigations (Figures 4.1 and 5.2) (Huang et al., 2009, Whitnall et al., 2008) and TEM studies (Figures 5.5A and B), the μ_{eff} of the mutant heart (2.17 ± 0.02 μ_B) demonstrates that iron is not being incorporated into ferritin, since the μ_{eff} of ferritin is 3.4 μ_B (Gutierrez et al., 2006).

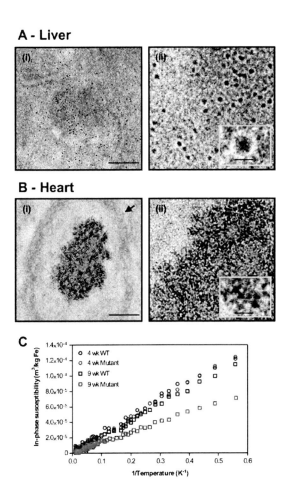

A - Liver

B - Heart

C

Figure 5.5 In the absence of frataxin, iron in the mutant heart accumulates as aggregates, markedly different in composition to that of ferritin which is observed in the frataxin-expressing liver of these animals. Transmission electron micrographs of unstained tissue from mutant mice at: **(i)** low and **(ii)** high magnification. **(A)** In the liver, iron appears in isolated, electron-dense, spherical ferritin particles (see inset) which are randomly distributed throughout the tissue. **(B)** In the heart, iron is observed in smaller, electron-dense, inter-connected particles (see inset), which coalesce into large, heterogeneous aggregates. Scale bars in Figures 5.5A and B are (i) 200nm; and (ii) inset 6 nm. **(C) From 4- to 9-weeks of age, iron accumulating in the mutant heart undergoes changes in magnetic susceptibility.** Hearts from 4- and 9-week-old WT and mutant mice were freeze dried, homogenised, and their magnetic susceptibility in an AC field was measured. The in-phase component of the AC magnetic susceptibility of 4- and 9-week-old WT and mutant mice is shown per mass of iron.

5.4 DISCUSSION

Friedreich's ataxia is a severe and debilitating disease caused by frataxin deficiency and is marked by the significant and toxic accumulation of iron within the mitochondria of the heart and neurons (Puccio et al., 2001, Richardson, 2003, Rötig et al., 1997, Rustin et al., 1999, Seznec et al., 2004, Velasco-Sanchez et al., 2010, Whitnall et al., 2008, Wong et al., 1999). Although the precise function of frataxin has not been defined, accumulating evidence suggests it acts as an iron chaperone for ISC synthesis (Leidgens et al., 2010, Richardson et al., 2010, Wang and Craig, 2008, Yoon and Cowan, 2003). Additional studies are required to fully elucidate the role of frataxin in iron metabolism, and will enable the development of new therapeutic regimes for the treatment of FA.

5.4.1 Cytosolic Iron Deficiency and the Effect of Iron Supplementation Using a High Iron Diet

In the frataxin mutant mouse heart, the existence of a cytosolic iron deficiency, in the face of mitochondrial iron loading (Whitnall et al., 2008), provides a target for therapeutic intervention within both cellular compartments. In Chapter 4 it was demonstrated that targeted removal of mitochondrial iron using the mitochondrial-permeable chelator PIH in combination with DFO, limits cardiomyopathy in the MCK mutant heart (Whitnall et al., 2008). In the current chapter, dietary iron supplementation was also demonstrated to limit cardiomyopathy in the MCK mutant heart (Figure 5.1B), though the reason for this was unclear. As IRP activity indicates cytosolic iron status (Li et al., 2008), the absence of any change in mutant IRP2 expression (Figure 5.2A) or activity (Figure 5.3) following

154

dietary iron supplementation, could indicate that iron loaded diet was not able to reconstitute the iron deficient cytosol, or that reconstitution was below detectable levels in this model of complete frataxin knockout in the cardiomyocyte.

It is of interest to note that the increased expression of myosin-binding genes   (*e.g., Myh7*) is considered a compensatory response to increase muscle contraction during cardiac failure (Abdelaziz et al., 2005, Rodriguez et al., 2007), and mutations in these genes gives rise to hypertrophic cardiomyopathy (Girolami et al., 2010, Hernandez et al., 2007). Interestingly, *Myh7* is up-regulated in response to dietary iron *in vivo* (Rodriguez et al., 2007). It is therefore possible that dietary iron supplementation enhanced the expression of myosin-binding genes as a mechanism to alleviate the cardiac hypertrophy in the mutant in this study.

In previous *in vitro* models of FA, iron supplementation has been beneficial. For example, addition of exogenous iron as hemin was demonstrated by Napoli *et al.* to rescue defects in ISC enzymes in a cellular model of frataxin knockdown (Napoli et al., 2007). Although it was not demonstrated, Napoli and colleagues suggested this may have been a consequence of hemin's ability to increase the pool of bioavailable iron (Napoli et al., 2007, Li et al., 2008). Furthermore, *in vitro* studies using FA patient lymphoblasts demonstrated that the iron donor, ferric ammonium citrate, up-regulated frataxin expression by increasing cytosolic iron levels (Li et al., 2008). Potentially, these data suggest that dietary iron may have more of a beneficial effect in models of partial, rather than complete knockout of frataxin from the cell.

Consideration must be given to the possibility that exogenous iron from a regime of iron supplementation may worsen the pathology of FA if it is not appropriately targeted to the appropriate molecular machinery. To address the compartmental misregulation of iron in FA, a combination of therapies that replenish the iron-deficient cytosol and chelate iron accumulating in the mitochondrion, would be optimal. Indeed, strategies which address iron mis-distribution, may be beneficial not only for the treatment of FA, but other conditions of mitochondrial iron accumulation with cytosolic iron deficiency, such as X-linked sideroblastic anaemia, neurodegeneration with brain iron accumulation and myopathy with ISCU deficiency (Kakhlon et al., 2010).

5.4.2 Conditional Frataxin Deletion in the Heart Leads to Systemic Alterations in Iron Metabolism

While frataxin interacts with *de novo* ISC assembly machinery, its exact molecular function still remains unclear (Pandolfo and Pastore, 2009). Our molecular work herein, recognises the marked differences that arise in the metabolism of iron *in vivo* as a result of frataxin deletion in the mutant heart, and in the mutant liver, where frataxin is intact. Despite dietary iron loading, the loss of frataxin expression in the mutant still leads to marked alterations in local cardiac iron metabolism as well as systemic processing of iron, and this reinforces the crucial role frataxin must play in iron metabolism (Richardson et al., 2010, Stemmler et al., 2010). Moreover, the increased levels of iron in the liver, spleen and kidney in the mutant, indicate that deletion of frataxin in the heart and skeletal muscle, causes an increase in systemic iron uptake and storage. This implies that the mutant heart is able to communicate its cytosolic iron deficiency and increased iron need systemically to other compartments within the body.

156

Intriguingly, we observed an inverse correlation between Hjv expression in the mutant heart (down-regulation compared to WT mice; Figure 5.2A) and mutant liver (up-regulation compared to WT mice; Figure 5.2B). This may have important implications with respect to the communicative pathways involved in iron signalling between the heart and liver. Indeed, while membrane-bound Hjv (mHjv) is known to act upstream of the key iron regulatory hormone, hepcidin, in the liver (Huang et al., 2005, Papanikolaou et al., 2004), little is known regarding the role of Hjv in the heart. This is surprising considering that Hjv expression in mammals is highest in the heart and skeletal muscle and lower in the liver (Papanikolaou et al., 2004, Zhang et al., 2007a). Under conditions of iron-deficiency, Hjv is cleaved and a soluble isoform (sHjv) is secreted (Lin et al., 2005, Silvestri et al., 2008, Zhang et al., 2007a). Although the cellular origin of sHjv is controversial, studies have ascertained that it represses the signal for hepcidin synthesis by binding to and antagonising mHjv (Lin et al., 2005, Babitt et al., 2007, Lin et al., 2008). Given current limitations in antibody specificity, the isoform of Hjv detected in Chapter 5 is unknown. Despite this, our observations in the mutant heart and liver, provide evidence to corroborate the hypothesis that the heart, as an iron- and energy-consuming organ, may utilize Hjv to regulate systemic iron metabolism and communicate its metabolic needs to the main iron storage organ, the liver (Hentze et al., 2010, Darshan and Anderson, 2009, Silvestri et al., 2008, Kuninger et al., 2006).

It is of interest that similar findings were recently reported in a mouse model of cardiac copper deficiency (Kim et al., 2010). Like iron, copper is a redox-active metal and an essential cofactor for metabolic functions *e.g.*, mitochondrial oxidative phosphorylation (Madsen and Gitlin, 2007, Kim et al., 2008). Conditional knockout of the cellular copper transporter molecule

1 (*Ctr1*) in murine cardiomyocytes, caused cardiac copper deficiency. In response to this, the heart activated a systemic signalling mechanism to communicate its increased metabolic need for copper to the liver, which is also a major copper store (Kim et al., 2010). While the serum proteins involved in these communicative pathways were not elucidated, this important study reinforces our findings that highlight the ability of the heart to initiate cross-organ communication of metal status. This is probably linked to the crucial role of the heart in maintaining circulation, and in the survival of the organism, and hence, its metabolic needs are of paramount importance in terms of continued functioning.

5.4.3 Iron Accumulation in the Mitochondrion of the Mutant Heart Does Not Occur as Ferritin

Studies in Chapter 4 previously demonstrated that frataxin knockout in the mutant heart increases uptake of cellular iron *via* TfR1 (Whitnall et al., 2008), with consequential targeting of iron to the mitochondrion giving rise to cytosolic iron deficiency, decreased cytosolic ferritin expression and mitochondrial iron overload (Whitnall et al., 2008). The present study demonstrates, on a visual basis using TEM, that cardiac iron within the mitochondrion of the mutant does not accumulate within a ferritin-like molecule, but most likely as a well crystallised, anti-ferromagnetic mineral iron aggregate of no defined structure (Figures 5.5A and B). This finding is in agreement with the molecular work in Chapter 4 (Whitnall et al., 2008) and in the current Chapter, in which demonstrated that ferritin is decreased in the mutant heart relative to the WT (Figure 5.2A). This work is in contrast to studies conducted by others, which suggests that iron is present in MIT ferritin in FA fibroblasts and cardiomyocytes (Michael et al., 2006, Popescu et al., 2007).

158

To further investigate the molecular nature of iron which accumulated within the mutant mitochondria, the magnetic properties of the tissue, which can provide information on the state of the iron present, were assessed. Magnetic susceptibility measurements demonstrated that the iron present within the heart of the mutant was not present as ferritin, but was consistent with a well crystallised mineral iron aggregate. This observation was strongly supported by our TEM studies that indicated that iron was not present in isolated spherical ferritin protein shells, but as smaller, irregularly shaped, inter-connected, electron-dense particles approximately 1 nm in diameter.

It is of interest that the iron aggregates observed in the mutant mitochondria of MCK mice (Figure 5.5B), were similar in appearance to haemosiderin (Allen et al., 2000, St Pierre et al., 1998). In iron loaded rat myocytes, haemosiderin appears under TEM as an insoluble heterogeneous aggregate composed of variable particle size, eletron density and magnetic susceptibility (Iancu, 1992). Haemosiderin is often found in pathological conditions of iron overload, and is thought that to be derived from the degradation of ferritin within the lysosome (Allen et al., 2000, St Pierre et al., 1998). Within haemosiderin, three different iron(III) oxyhydroxide structures have been identified that show similarities to: (i) the mineral ferrihydrite; (ii) poorly crystalline goethite; and (iii) a non-crystalline iron(III) oxyhydroxide particle (Hackett et al., 2007). The ferrihydrite-like form of haemosiderin may be more toxic and easier to chelate than the goethite-like form (St Pierre et al., 1998), and chelator combinations are able to remove excess haemosiderin iron from mutant cardiomyocytes (Whitnall et al., 2008). Considering this, further analysis is required to fully identify the precise chemical species contained within mutant mitochondrial iron aggregates. Regardless of this, it is evident from our studies, that without the proposed iron chaperone (Yoon and Cowan, 2003, Richardson et al., 2010, Wang and Craig, 2008, Leidgens et al., 2010, Yoon and Cowan, 2004, Lesuisse et al., 2003, Schoenfeld et al., 2005, Zhang et al., 2005b) or detoxification (Richardson et al., 2010, O'Neill et al., 2005) functions of frataxin, iron that should be incorporated into ISCs, MIT ferritin, or haem, is instead depositing as small, well crystallized inorganic particles that are distinct from ferritin.

In conclusion, this study demonstrates that dietary iron supplementation may be of benefit in the treatment of FA. It also underlines the previously unidentified systemic changes that occur as a result of frataxin deletion in the MCK mutant heart. The results indicate that deletion of frataxin not only directly affects the iron metabolism of the targeted organ (*e.g.*, the heart), but also markedly influences systemic iron metabolism. Indeed, it is thought that systemic signalling leads to a rescue response in order to correct the cytosolic iron deficiency of the heart. These studies demonstrate the key role of the heart and its role in regulating systemic iron metabolism. Furthermore, mitochondrial iron which accumulates consequential to the loss of frataxin in the mutant heart, is present in well crystallised mineral aggregates that are distinct from ferritin.

CHAPTER 6
GENERAL DISCUSSION AND FUTURE
DIRECTIONS

6.1 DISCUSSION PRELUDE

Strong evidence demonstrates that iron plays critical functions that are indispensible for life (Rouault and Tong, 2008, Sheftel and Lill, 2009). At the beginning of my PhD candidature, much research had already been performed to examine the many pathways and proteins that traffic iron and regulate its utilisation (Levi and Rovida, 2009). Indeed, many of these mechanisms were deciphered through the analysis of animal models that mimic human disease. When these regulatory mechanisms fail and lead to iron overload or deficiency, or are exploited for the benefit of the neoplastic cell, therapies that target iron can potentially be implemented (Kalinowski and Richardson, 2005). To this extent, the studies in this thesis examine novel iron chelators for the treatment of cancer. They also assess iron chelation and iron supplementation strategies for the treatment of FA, and dissect the iron trafficking pathways in this disease.

Specifically, data in Chapter 3 highlight the significant and selective anti-tumour activity of the novel iron chelator, Dp44mT (Whitnall et al., 2006). Results in Chapter 4 began to identify the pathways that cause mitochondrial iron loading in the severe neuro- and cardio-degenerative disease, FA, and indicate the therapeutic benefit that could be gained if mitochondrial-permeable iron chelators such as PIH are used to treat cardiac pathology in FA (Whitnall et al., 2008). Studies in Chapter 5 and the future investigations discussed below, indicate why iron supplementation may also be an option for treating the cytosolic iron deficiency observed in FA. Moreover, the findings in this latter chapter also demonstrate the potential influence of the heart on systemic iron metabolism, and may represent a new paradigm in iron metabolism.

6.2 A CLASS OF IRON CHELATORS WITH A WIDE SPECTRUM OF POTENT ANTI-TUMOUR ACTIVITY THAT OVERCOME RESISTANCE TO CHEMOTHERAPEUTICS

6.2.1 Significance and Summary of Principal Findings - Chapter 3

Cancer is the leading cause of death worldwide and the total number of cases globally is increasing (WHO, 2008). Moreover, multi-drug resistance and non-specific anti-tumour drug toxicity complicate established therapies (Grahame-Smith and Aronson, 2006, Schneider et al., 1994). Consequently, new anti-cancer therapeutics with novel mechanisms of action are required. Neoplastic cells are metabolically more active than their normal counterparts and thus metabolic inhibitors represent an important class of anti-tumour agents. Iron chelators in particular have gained recent attention, owing to their ability to retard DNA synthesis by limiting iron availability for the rate-limiting step in this pathway, ribonucleotide reductase (Finch et al., 2000). In addition, these agents also affect the expression of molecules that regulate the cell cycle such as p53, GADD45, cyclins D1, D2 and D3, p21 and CDK2 (Chaston et al., 2003, Darnell and Richardson, 1999, Gao and Richardson, 2001, Nurtjahja-Tjendraputra et al., 2007). The multiple effects of chelators on molecules involved in DNA synthesis and cell cycle progression, leads to G_1/S cell cycle arrest and apoptosis (Richardson et al., 2009).

Considering the important potential role of chelators as anti-cancer agents, the studies in Chapter 3 extensively examined a suite of novel DpT and PKIH iron chelator analogues, to identify potential candidates for *in vivo* anti-tumour testing. Based on the average IC_{50} across 28 cell types tested, all DpT chelators and some PKIH analogues exhibited high anti-proliferative activity. Importantly, this activity was: (i) markedly greater than that of the clinically used iron chelator, DFO; (ii) equal or greater than that of the clinically-trialled chelator, Triapine; and (iii) equal or greater than that of the clinically used anti-tumour anthracycline, DOX (Table 3.2) (Whitnall et al., 2006). Since mutation or functional inactivation of the tumour suppressor, p53, is a common feature of human tumours (Goh et al., 2011), it was important that for all examined chelators, no correlation was observed between IC_{50} and p53 status. This demonstrates that the activity of these agents does not depend on functional p53 and is an important criterion to enable broad anti-tumour efficacy in cancers with either mutant or wild-type p53. Collectively, these results indicated the potential of the DpT analogues in particular, for future therapeutic development against a diverse range of human tumours.

Amongst the tested chelators, Dp44mT exhibited the greatest anti-proliferative activity and was considerably more effective than DFO, Triapine and DOX. For this reason, the anti-tumour profile of Dp44mT was investigated in detail. Importantly, Dp44mT was able to overcome multi-drug resistance mechanisms of etoposide-resistant MCF-7/VP breast cancer cells and vinblastine-resistant KB-V1 epidermoid carcinoma cells (Figure 3.2) (Whitnall et al., 2006). The significance of this finding is that drug resistance against a variety of common anti-cancer agents is a serious problem in the clinics, and thus agents that can overcome this, such as Dp44mT, are vital to develop.

The potent *in vitro* efficacy of Dp44mT was mirrored *in vivo* in a range of human tumour xenografts in nude mice (Figure 3.3) (Whitnall et al., 2006). After short- and long-term administration, tumour growth in Dp44mT treated mice was markedly inhibited in comparison to the vehicle-treated controls. As a clinical comparison over short-term studies, Dp44mT, at over a 16-fold lower dose (0.75mg/kg/day), showed significantly greater *in vivo* anti-tumour activity than the clinically trialled chelator, Triapine (12mg/kg/day). Importantly, Dp44mT did not cause overt body iron depletion, nor were there any alterations observed in most haematological or biochemical indices. Unfortunately, Dp44mT did cause dose-dependent cardiac fibrosis, which can be speculated to be due to its marked redox activity (Figure 3.4) (Whitnall et al., 2006). However, the precise molecular mechanism of this toxicological effect remains unknown (Richardson et al., 2006, Yuan et al., 2004). If Dp44mT were to be considered for clinical development, this side effect would clearly need to be addressed.

Interestingly, Dp44mT up-regulated the expression of the tumour growth and metastasis suppressor *NDRG1* in the tumour, but not the liver (Figure 3.5) (Whitnall et al., 2006). This indicates a potential mechanism of selective anti-cancer activity that could prevent metastasis, which may be of particular importance in the treatment of many aggressive tumours (Kovacevic et al., 2008), when metastasis often determines the fate of the patient.

6.2.2 Subsequent Studies and Future Experiments Examining the Development of Iron Chelators as Cancer Therapeutics

6.2.2.1 The Anti-Metastatic Effect of Dp44mT

As introduced briefly above, metastatic disease is a significant clinical problem, as demonstrated by the high number (approximately 90%) of cancer-related deaths which result from metastasis (Tse and Kalluri, 2007, Yoshida et al., 2000). Recent research has demonstrated that NDRG1 up-regulation plays a critical role in preventing metastasis, and a strong correlation has been found between NDRG1 expression and patient prognosis, particularly in prostate and breast cancer patients (Bandyopadhyay et al., 2003, Bandyopadhyay et al., 2004a, Bandyopadhyay et al., 2004b). Considering this, it was important that Dp44mT exhibited potent anti-tumour activity against breast and prostate cancer cell lines *in vitro* (Table 3.2) and up-regulated *NDRG1 in vivo* (Figure 3.5) (Whitnall et al., 2006). To directly determine if Dp44mT inhibits metastasis *in vivo*, a model of tumour metastasis could be used, such as the AT6.1 spontaneous lung metastasis model (Bandyopadhyay et al., 2003), or the Lewis lung carcinoma model (Funakoshi et al., 2000, Hatakawa et al., 2002). After subcutaneous injection (Bandyopadhyay et al., 2003) or surgical implantation (Funakoshi et al., 2000, Hatakawa et al., 2002) of the tumour into the flank of mice, tumours metastasise to the lung and the degree of severity can be quantified by macroscopic examination (Bandyopadhyay et al., 2003) or fluorescence microscopy (Funakoshi et al., 2000, Hatakawa et al., 2002), respectively. This would identify the ability of Dp44mT treatment to prevent tumour metastasis from the primary site of inoculation *in vivo*.

Angiogenesis also plays an integral role in the persistence of primary solid tumours and their metastasis. The metastasis models proposed above could also be used to indicate the extent to which tumour metastasis is affected by the competing signals of *NDRG1* up-regulation and up-regulation of the pro-angiogenic factor *VEGF1*, which were observed *in vivo* after Dp44mT treatment (Figure 3.5) (Whitnall et al., 2006). Both VEGF1 and NDRG1 are HIF-1α targets and their expression can be transcriptionally up-regulated by iron-depletion (Chong et al., 2002, Hagist et al., 2009, Le and Richardson, 2004, Linden et al., 2003, Zhang et al., 2007b). To this end, immunohistochemical staining using antibodies against the endothelial marker, CD34 (DAKO, Glostrup, Denmark), could be performed on primary tumours from Chapter 3, and the primary and metastatic tumours from the aforementioned metastatic models. This would quantify microvessel density and examine the effect of Dp44mT on tumour vascularisation (Guşet et al., 2010). At the same time, expression of both *VEGF1* and *NDRG1* could be assessed in these tumours by RT-PCR methods described in Section 3.2.7. In comparison, CD34 staining, *VEGF1* and *NDRG1* expression could also be examined in healthy tissues *e.g.,* liver, brain, kidney *etc*, to investigate the effect of iron chelation on angiogenesis, metastasis and healthy tissue vasculature in the metastatic models.

6.2.2.2 New Mechanisms of Action Justify Further Development of Dp44mT

Subsequent studies have confirmed that in addition to its iron-binding activity, redox-related oxidative stress generated by the Dp44mT-Fe and/or Dp44mT-Cu complexes is also an important factor in the anti-proliferative efficacy of Dp44mT (Bendova et al., 2010, Jansson et al., 2010, Kalinowski et al., 2007, Mladenka et al., 2009, Richardson et al., 2006). This bimodal mechanism by which Dp44mT acts, has been described as the "double-punch effect" (Kalinowski and Richardson, 2007). As possible secondary mechanisms to the double-punch effect, Dp44mT has recently been demonstrated to: (i) inhibit DNA topoisomerase-2α and induce DNA strand breaks (Rao et al., 2009); (ii) induce apoptosis by interfering with mitochondrial membrane potential and causing caspase-3 activation (Noulsri et al., 2009); and (iii) similarly to other iron chelators, Dp44mT induces G_1/S arrest (Noulsri et al., 2009). These observations add to the previously identified ability of Dp44mT to induce apoptosis by decreasing the ratio of anti-apoptotic Bcl-2 to pro-apoptotic Bax, releasing mitochondrial cytochrome c (Yuan et al., 2004) and up-regulating NDRG1 *in vitro* (Le and Richardson, 2004) and *in vivo* (Figure 3.5) (Whitnall et al., 2006).

Collectively, the results above highlight the multi-faceted effects which underlie the potent anti-tumour activity of Dp44mT and may explain its ability to overcome drug resistance to other chemotherapeutics and act independently of p53 status (Whitnall et al., 2006). They also justify why this novel and patented compound should be considered for pharmacokinetic studies which precede clinical development.

6.2.2.3 Pharmacokinetic Studies

Recently developed high-performance liquid chromatography (HPLC) methods have demonstrated the stability of Dp44mT and investigated its breakdown products in rabbit and human plasma, *in vitro*, over a 24 h time period (Stariat et al., 2009). Based on these preliminary studies, these HPLC methods could potentially be used to assess the stability of Dp44mT in plasma *in vivo*. To do this, Dp44mT could be administered to a cohort of healthy nude mice as described in Section 3.2.5. At time intervals (*e.g.*, between 15 min - 24 h) post i.v. injection, mice could then be progressively culled, blood collected *via* cardiac puncture, and serum separated as per Section 3.2.6 for HPLC analysis.

The biodistribution and metabolism of Dp44mT could also be examined by labelling Dp44mT with ^{14}C (Allemann et al., 1994, Coldham et al., 2002, Wiegand et al., 2002). Commercially labelled ^{14}C-Dp44mT (Izotop, Budapest, Hungary) could be administered to xenografted nude mice using treatment regimes described in Section 3.2.5. Faeces and urine could be collected *via* the use of metabolic cages (Wong et al., 2004), and the heart, liver, spleen, kidney, tumour and brain harvested. After sample combustion, the level of ^{14}C in these specimens could then be measured by β-scintillation counting (Wiegand et al., 2002). Evidence of ^{14}C in the brain would indicate the ability of Dp44mT to permeate the blood-brain barrier, which may be important for the treatment of neurological tumours. To assess the generation of Dp44mT metabolites in tissues and faeces, homogenates could be extracted with acetonitrile under acidic conditions, after which protein precipitation could be carried out by centrifugation (Wiegand et al., 2002). The collected supernatant could then be analysed by HPLC, measured for ^{14}C levels (Wiegand et al., 2002) in relation to previous studies where Dp44mT metabolites were observed *in vitro* and compared to the previously identified metabolite profile of Dp44mT in plasma *in vitro* (Stariat et al., 2009).

With increased knowledge of the pharmacological profile and metabolism of Dp44mT *in vivo*, the frequency of administration could potentially be re-optimised, and this may alleviate cardiac fibrosis. Indeed in the current work, the doses of Dp44mT used were based on short-term maximum tolerated dose studies (Yuan et al., 2004) and were not extensively optimised for long-term experiments (Whitnall et al., 2006). Hence, this may partly explain some of the toxicological effects observed.

6.2.2.4 Structure-Activity Analysis of Dp44mT

Importantly, for the first time, my studies have illustrated the anti-tumour potency of the general DpT structure *in vivo* using human tumours in nude mice. Based on the pronounced activity of these ligands, structurally similar iron chelators have since been developed in our laboratory (Kalinowski et al., 2007, Richardson et al., 2006). Indeed, this was done to achieve a more favourable balance between efficacy and toxicity, and to circumvent the cardiac fibrosis associated with Dp44mT. An iron chelator with soft electron donors such as nitrogen and sulfur, enhances the production of ROS after complexation with iron (Kalinowski et al., 2007, Yu et al., 2009). Therefore, molecular modifications have largely focused on retaining these groups in order to preserve their ability to redox cycle and induce anti-proliferative effects, while making structural changes elsewhere in the molecule to alter lipophilicity and electron-donating/withdrawing substituents.

The first structural modification made to the basic DpT backbone structure (Figure 6.1A), has been the addition of a phenyl ring (circled, Figure 6.1B) in place of the non-coordinating 2-pyridyl group (circled, Figure 6.1A) found in DpT analogues. The resulting 2-benzoylpyridine thiosemicarbazone (BpT) analogues (Figure 6.1B) are more lipophilic and their lower redox potentials make the BpT-Fe complexes more redox active than their DpT counterparts (Kalinowski et al., 2007, Richardson et al., 2006). Studies are currently underway to assess the *in vivo* efficacy of these BpT chelators (Richardson et al., 2009).

The potent anti-proliferative activity of Dp44mT in comparison to other DpT analogues (Chapter 3) (Whitnall et al., 2006, Yuan et al., 2004), may be correlated to the unique structure of this ligand. Of all DpT analogues, Dp44mT is the only compound without hydrogen groups bound to the terminal nitrogen atom at position 4 (Figure 3.1). Considering this, a second potential structural modification of Dp44mT could substitute the terminal hydrogen group in Dp4aT, Dp4eT and Dp4pt, with an extra allyl, ethyl or phenyl group, respectively. The generated analogues could then be screened using the MTT assay described in Section 3.2.3 to determine their

170

in vitro anti-tumour efficacy, using Dp44mT and DFO as positive controls (Whitnall et al., 2006).

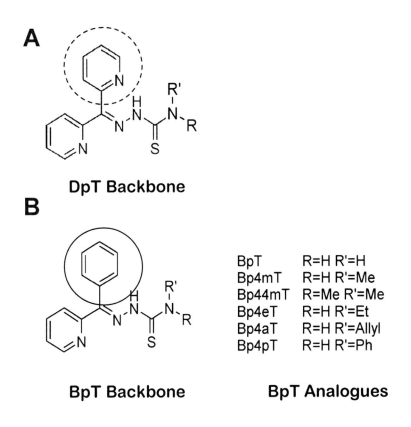

Figure 6.1 Structural modification made to the backbone of DpT to produce the BpT backbone structure and more lipophilic BpT analogues. (A) Replacement of the non-coordinating 2-pyridyl group (dashed blue circle) in the DpT backbone with a **(B)** phenyl ring (solid blue circle) to produce the BpT backbone and BpT analogues. Adapted from (Yu et al., 2009).

6.3 CONDITIONAL FRATAXIN KNOCKOUT IN THE FRIEDREICH'S ATAXIA HEART: TREATMENT BY IRON CHELATION THERAPY AND ELUCIDATION OF MITOCHONDRIAL IRON LOADING PATHWAYS

6.3.1 Significance and Summary of Principal Findings - Chapter 4

The clinical symptoms and hereditary nature of FA were first described over a century ago (Friedreich, 1863c, Friedreich, 1863b, Friedreich, 1863a, Friedreich, 1876, Friedreich, 1877, Harding, 1981, Ladame, 1890). Yet the identification of myocardial iron deposits (Ladame, 1890, Sanchez-Casis et al., 1976), their concomitant mitochondrial location (Foury and Cazzalini, 1997, Puccio et al., 2001) and contribution to FA pathogenesis (Foury and Cazzalini, 1997, Radisky et al., 1999, Rötig et al., 1997, Rustin et al., 1999, Wong et al., 1999), were not described until much later. Until the studies undertaken in Chapter 4, the molecular mechanisms responsible for the cardiac mitochondrial iron accumulation in the absence of frataxin had not been defined.

The findings in Chapter 4 clearly demonstrated that frataxin deficiency increases cellular iron uptake *via* TfR1, with consequential targeting of iron to the mitochondrion causing accumulation of mitochondrial iron that is not being: (i) used for synthesis of the ISC-containing protein SDHA; nor (ii) sequestered by MIT ferritin (Chapter 4) (Whitnall et al., 2008). In subsequent studies from our laboratory (Huang et al., 2009) which also used the MCK mutant mouse, additional deficiencies were identified in ISC and haem synthetic pathway proteins themselves. These included the ISC assembly protein, Iscu1/2, and the haem synthetic pathway proteins, Fech, 5-aminolevulinate dehydratase and uroporphyrinogen III synthase (Huang et al., 2009). Of relevance, mitochondrial iron does not accumulate to a

172

significant level until 7 weeks of age in the MCK mutant mouse (Puccio et al., 2001), while the aforementioned deficiencies in Iscu1/2 and Fech were detected at 4 weeks of age (Huang et al., 2009). Taken together, these results in addition to my studies in Chapter 4, are clear indications of how iron accumulates within the mitochondrion, given that iron entering this organelle is not being sequestered into MIT ferritin or effectively used in the ISC and haem biosynthetic pathways.

In contrast to the mitochondrial iron-loading described above, my studies also identified the presence of a cytosolic iron-deficiency (Chapter 4) (Whitnall et al., 2008). This finding was based on experimental data which directly demonstrated that in the heart there was: (i) a decreased proportion of cytosolic iron; (ii) decreased expression of the cytosolic storage proteins, L- and H-ferritin; and (iii) increased IRP2-RNA binding activity (Chapter 4) (Whitnall et al., 2008). Similarly, Li and colleagues also demonstrated that IRP2 protein expression and RNA-binding activity were increased in FA patient lymphoblasts (Li et al., 2008). Considering this, it is of critical importance that the iron metabolism pathways involved in FA pathogenesis are fully understood, as this could identify novel therapeutic strategies. Indeed, the identification of the cytosolic iron deficiency in the MCK mutant was the premise on which dietary iron loading experiments in Chapter 5 were based.

Importantly, the studies in Chapter 4 were the first to conclusively demonstrate that iron chelators can remove toxic accumulations of iron and limit FA cardiac hypertrophy *in vivo* (Whitnall et al., 2008). The mitochondrion-permeable chelator, PIH, in combination with the extracellular ligand, DFO (Link et al., 2003), decreased cardiac iron in the MCK mutant to levels that were comparable to WT mice without causing overt cardiac iron-depletion. Importantly, chelation therapy also limited cardiac hypertrophy in this severe MCK model of FA cardiomyopathy (Figure 4.4) (Whitnall et al., 2008).

Although treatment of MCK mutant mice with PIH and DFO did not benefit animal growth or restore SDHA expression (Figure 4.4) (Whitnall et al., 2008), this does not detract from the value that iron chelation therapy may have in FA. Cardiomyopathy is the leading cause of death in FA patients (Delatycki et al., 2000), and currently there are no effective treatments available for this condition. The development of new therapeutic strategies is therefore an urgent issue. Removal of mitochondrial iron accumulation is key to the success of iron chelation therapy in FA, as it hinders the participation of iron in ROS-mediated cytotoxicity (Lim et al., 2008, Richardson, 2003). Phase II clinical trials are currently examining the use of the chelator, deferiprone, for the treatment of FA (Santos et al., 2010). However, the toxicity of this drug remains controversial, particularly considering its haematological side effects, such as severe agranulocytosis (Piga et al., 2010). In comparison, using the MCK mouse model, PIH and DFO did not affect the haematological parameters or histology of major organs (Chatper 4) (Whitnall et al., 2008). As discussed in Section 4.4, it is anticipated that PIH alone would suffice for treatment in a clinical setting, since human FA is far less aggressive than the pathology observed in the MCK mutant mouse model (Puccio et al., 2001, Whitnall et al., 2008). The studies in this thesis indicate that PIH may be a safe and viable therapeutic option to deferiprone, if administration of a chelator to FA patients is deemed appropriate and useful.

6.3.2 Future Studies Examining Intracellular Iron Trafficking Pathways in the MCK Mouse

While significant changes were demonstrated in the intracellular iron trafficking pathways in MCK mice (Chapter 4) (Whitnall et al., 2008), further studies are required before they can be fully dissected. In addition to elucidating possible therapeutic options, this would also add value to current knowledge regarding iron metabolism in general, and may also help to elucidate the precise function of frataxin in iron homeostasis.

6.3.2.1 Cellular Iron Uptake

Although studies presented in this thesis demonstrate significant uptake of iron *via* the classical Tf-TfR1 pathway (Figure 4.1), uptake of non-transferrin bound iron (NTBI) was not explored. A major source of pathological tissue iron accumulation in patients with systemic iron overload is NTBI (Cabantchik et al., 2005), which may enter cells by unregulated routes (Glickstein et al., 2006) and can affect cardiac function (Shvartsman et al., 2007). At this stage, it is unclear if the MCK model or FA patients have significant levels of circulating NTBI. However, considering the marked systemic alterations in iron metabolism in the MCK mouse and iron loading of the liver and spleen (Chapter 5), it is possible that NTBI could be present and is worth investigating.

The precise chemical form of iron which constitutes plasma NTBI has been difficult to define (Anderson and Vulpe, 2009) and large variations in serum NTBI measurements have been described between different methods of detection (Kolb et al., 2009). Furthermore, the distribution of NTBI into subcellular organelles has not been well researched and methods are not comprehensive (Shvartsman et al., 2007). A suitable initial means of ascertaining whether NTBI plays a role in the MCK model of FA would be to measure serum indices such as serum iron concentration (*i.e.,* Tf-bound-iron) and unbound iron-binding capacity (UIBC). This can be routinely done *via* colourimetric analysis using a Konelab 20i analyser (Thermo Electron Corporation). From this, calculations can be made of total iron-binding capacity (TIBC; TIBC = serum iron + UIBC) and Tf-saturation (serum iron/TIBC x 100) (Dunn et al., 2006). Although serum iron has been measured in FA patients previously, the cohort assessed was extremely small (*n* = 10 patients) (Wilson et al., 1998) and more statistically sound evaluation is required. If iron is present in excess of Tf-saturation and TIBC, this could denote that NTBI is present. On the basis of these results and in the advent of more accurate methods to investigate intracellular NTBI trafficking, it may then be feasible to test the hypothesis of Shvartsman and colleagues, namely, that mitochondria rapidly acquire NTBI as a mechanism that leads to surplus iron accumulation in this organelle and in FA (Shvartsman et al., 2007). Additionally, investigations into serum iron indices would complement future studies examining systemic iron overload in the MCK mutant and in FA (Section 6.4.3).

6.3.2.2 Cytosolic Iron Transporters

The increased 'need' for iron in MCK mutant cardiac mitochondria is reminiscent of the high iron requirements which are required for haemoglobin synthesis in mitochondria of reticulocytes (Richardson et al., 1996). In light of this, experiments could be performed to examine if MCK mutants use the reticulocyte 'kiss and run' mechanism to deliver iron directly from Tf-containing endosomes to mitochondria (Sheftel et al., 2007). This pathway by-passes the cytosol (Sheftel et al., 2007) and could be facilitated by the mammalian exocyst protein, Sec15l1 (Sheftel et al., 2007, Zhang et al., 2006a). Observations of cytosolic iron deficiency

(Whitnall et al., 2008) and increased Sec15l1 protein expression in MCK mutants (Huang et al., 2009), strengthens the possibility that a 'kiss and run' mechanism may exist in this model. Briefly, studies would entail harvesting neonatal cardiomyocytes from WT and MCK mutant mice using established procedures in our laboratory (Kwok and Richardson, 2002, Kwok and Richardson, 2004), and labelling mitochondria with Mitotracker CMXRos (Molecular Probes, Eugene, USA). Fluorescently labelled Tf (Alexa Green 488 Tf; Molecular Probes) would then be added to the cardiomyocyte culture and Tf-endosomal movement recorded under a confocal microscope as described by Sheftel and colleagues (Sheftel et al., 2007). The co-localisation of red-stained mitochondria and green-stained Tf-containing endosomes could then be assessed using Image analysis software (Metamorph™, Molecular Devices, Sunnyvale, USA) to quantify and differentiate endosomal-mitochondrial contact in WT and mutant mice (Sheftel et al., 2007).

Examination of the endocytosis of Tf could also be performed using Tf labeled with ^{125}I (PerkinElmer) and ^{59}Fe. This would allow us to track the intracellular trafficking of Tf bound with ^{125}I following endocytosis in cardiomyocytes derived from the MCK mutant mice compared to their WT counterparts. Standard methods in our laboratory would be used to label Tf with ^{59}Fe and ^{125}I (Richardson and Baker, 1990, Richardson and Baker, 1992) and to prepare primary cardiomyocyte cultures (Kwok and Richardson, 2002, Kwok and Richardson, 2004). The alterations in the rate of endocytosis of ^{125}I-Tf and the intracellular distribution of the label in terms of the percentage of ^{125}I-Tf internalised would be assessed using standard methods (Richardson and Baker, 1990, Richardson and Baker, 1992). The intracellular distribution of ^{125}I-Tf in subcellular compartments could also be investigated using the methods described in Section 4.2.6 to produce cytosolic and SMM fractions.

A cytosolic iron chaperone that delivers iron to ferritin was recently identified in yeast (Shi et al., 2008). Human poly (rC)-binding protein 1 (PCBP1) is an RNA-binding protein that is ubiquitously expressed in mammalian cells in the cytosol and nucleus (Makeyev and Liebhaber, 2002). Cytosolic metallo-chaperones which deliver metals to their cognate enzymes and transporters have been identified for nickel and copper (Kuchar and Hausinger, 2004, O'Halloran and Culotta, 2000, Pufahl et al., 1997, Rae et al., 1999). Considering the numerous iron-dependent enzymes in the cytosol, it would be expected that iron should similarly possess a cytosolic chaperone, that would mirror the role of frataxin acting as a chaperone for mitochondrial ISC synthesis (Shi et al., 2008). In a yeast cell model, PCBP1 bound to ferritin, and using human cells *in vitro*, depletion of PCPB1 inhibited ferritin iron-loading (Shi et al., 2008). As an extension of this, it would be interesting to examine protein expression of PCBP1 in MCK cardiac tissue, given that expression of cytosolic H- and L- ferritin are decreased in the MCK mutant (Figure 4.1) (Whitnall et al., 2008). This could easily be performed *via* western blotting (Section 2.5) using the commercially available antibody from Abcam (Cambridge, USA) (Li et al., 2010).

6.3.2.3 Mitochondrial Iron Import

To complete an analysis of intracellular iron trafficking pathways, mitochondrial iron importers must be identified. Gene array data and RT-PCR have demonstrated that the mitochondrial iron transporter, mitoferrin2 (Mtfrn2), is up-regulated in the MCK mutant as early as 4 weeks of age (Huang et al., 2009). However at the time of publication (Huang et al., 2009), antibodies were not available to confirm these changes at the protein level. A Mtfrn2 antibody has since been prepared (Paradkar et al., 2009). Using this antibody, western blotting (Section 2.5) could be performed to determine if up-regulation of *Mtfrn2* mRNA translates into increased protein levels of this molecule. This would allow us to confirm if Mtfrn2 has a role in the pathway of mitochondrial iron accumulation in the MCK mouse.

6.3.3 Future Studies Examining Chelation Therapy in the MCK Mouse

6.3.3.1 Proof of Principle - Ensuring PIH Does Not Deplete the Cytosolic Compartment

Although it was not demonstrated directly, it was presumed that the PIH/DFO chelator combination was successful in removing iron deposits from the mitochondrion, as histological quantification of Prussian blue staining and ICP-AES measurements of cardiac iron concentration, both indicated that net cardiac iron levels were significantly reduced in the MCK mutant to normal WT levels (Figure 4.4) (Whitnall et al., 2008). Furthermore, the ability of PIH to permeate mitochondrial membranes and bind intra-mitochondrial iron accumulations has previously been demonstrated (Ponka et al., 1979a, Richardson et al., 2001). However, to confirm this chelator combination was not depleting the cytosolic compartment, which would exacerbate the cytosolic iron deficiency, IRP2-RNA binding activity assays could be performed using the methodology in Section 2.6 following PIH/DFO treatment of animals as per Section 4.2.3. An increase in IRP2-RNA binding in chelator- compared to control-treated mutants, would indicate that the cytosol was being further deprived of iron.

179

6.3.3.2 Analogues of 2-Pyridylcarboxaldehyde Isonicotinoyl Hydrazone (PCIH) as Ligands for the Treatment of Friedreich's Ataxia

A variety of studies *in vitro*, *in vivo* and in a clinical trial have demonstrated the potential of PIH for the treatment of iron overload disease (Brittenham, 1990, Cikrt et al., 1980, Hoy et al., 1979, Ponka et al., 1979a, Ponka et al., 1979b). Although unfortunately, PIH has been of little interest to the pharmaceutical industry, given that results on this promising chelator were published before patent protection was established (Richardson and Ponka, 1998). In light of this, a new series of tridentate ligands based on the structure of PIH have been synthesised and patented (Becker and Richardson, 1999). These ligands, known as the 2-pyridylcardoxyaldehyde isonicotinoyl hydrazone (PCIH) analogues (Figure 6.2), were produced in a similar fashion to PIH, *i.e.*, using a one-step Schiff base condensation reaction (Becker and Richardson, 1999). This would allow them to be economically produced on a commercial scale (Richardson, 2003).

Of the PCIH analogues, the following characteristics highlight why 2-pyridylcarboxaldehyde 2-thiophenecarboxyl hydrazone (PCTH; Figure 6.2) would be a suitable patent protected chelator to test in the MCK model of FA. In comparison to PIH, PCTH has: (i) similar *in vitro* iron chelation efficacy (Becker and Richardson, 1999); (ii) greater *in vitro* efficacy to rescue normal and FA fibroblasts from H_2O_2-mediated cytotoxicity, which is equal to that of the clinically trialled anti-oxidant, idebenone (Lim et al., 2008); (iii) similar lipophilicity (Becker and Richardson, 1999); (iv) similar ability to actively mobilise mitochondrial iron in an *in vitro* model of mitochondrial iron overload (Richardson et al., 2001); (v) comparable iron chelation efficacy in an *in vivo* rodent model of iron overload (Wong et al., 2004); and is (vi) orally active and well tolerated at optimal doses (Wong et al., 2004).

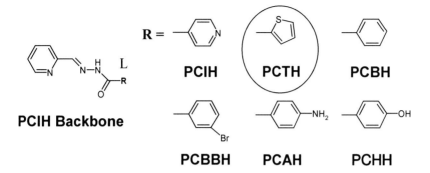

PCIH Backbone

PCIH PCTH PCBH

PCBBH PCAH PCHH

Figure 6.2 Structure of the PCIH chelator backbone and the derived PCIH analogues. One of the most potent ligands as demonstrated from *in vitro* studies, was PCTH (circled). Adapted from (Whitnall and Richardson, 2006)

In contrast to the requirements of anti-cancer chelators (Kalinowski and Richardson, 2005), ideal ligands for the treatment of iron overload *e.g.,* FA, must not exhibit marked redox activity or anti-proliferative activity. To this extent, it was important that PCTH had the following favourable properties, namely: (i) low *in vitro* anti-proliferative activity (Becker and Richardson, 1999); (ii) no marked effect on up-regulating the cell cycle arrest genes, *WAF1* and *GADD45* (Becker and Richardson, 1999); (iii) little redox activity (Chaston and Richardson, 2003a); and significantly (iv) it did not damage DNA in intact mammalian cells *in vitro* (Chaston and Richardson, 2003a).

Given these characteristics, PCTH would be a potential candidate for future development for the treatment of FA. In keeping with good ethical practice, a maximum tolerated dose study should first be performed to determine the optimal dose of PCTH, (which could be used in combination with DFO), for treatment of the MCK mouse. Based on the doses used in Section 4.2.3, and the similarities in efficacy when equal concentrations of PCTH and PIH are used *in vitro* (Becker and Richardson, 1999, Richardson et al., 2001) and *in vivo* (Wong et al., 2004), initial experiments could begin with doses of 50, 150 and 200 mg/kg/day of PCTH/DFO. Throughout the study, animals would be monitored for signs of discomfort and general malaise, their weight checked twice weekly and a battery of biological parameters such as haematology, histology, and serum biochemistry would be analysed using methods in Sections 2.3.1, 2.3.3 and 3.2.6, respectively. Once a maximum tolerated dose had been identified, experiments could then be carried out to test the efficacy and tolerability of PCTH/DFO in the MCK model following the methods and parameters assessed in Chapter 4.

6.3.4 Future Studies Examining Neurodegeneration in Friedreich's Ataxia

While cardiomyopathy is the leading cause of death in FA patients (Delatycki et al., 2000), neurodegeneration also has a significant impact on patient morbidity, causing ataxia and other neurological-associated symptoms (Santos et al., 2010). Like the cardiodegeneration observed in FA, mitochondrial damage, iron accumulation and ISC deficiencies also occur in the nervous system (Sturm et al., 2005). Addressing changes in neuropathology is an avenue that was not explored in the current thesis, and hence, future investigations require the examination of neuronal mouse models of FA.

6.3.4.1 The Neuron-Specific Enolase Transgenic Mouse Model

A number of mouse models exist for the *in vivo* study of FA (Puccio, 2009). Most pertinent of these is the neuron-specific enolase (NSE) model, which was developed in conjunction with the MCK mouse (Puccio et al., 2001). Frataxin deletion in the NSE mouse is under the control of the neuron-specific enolase promoter (hence the abbreviation, NSE), that induces tissue-specific deletion of frataxin in neurons (Puccio et al., 2001). In line with the human disease, the deletion of frataxin produces a neurological phenotype highlighted by ataxia, loss of proprioception and degeneration of the brainstem and cerebellum (Puccio et al., 2001). Surprisingly though, at the time of generating the NSE model, Puccio and colleagues did not indicate if brain iron accumulation was examined (Puccio et al., 2001). This is despite their more extensive investigations that examined iron accumulation in the MCK heart and mitochondrion using electron microscopy and histological staining (Puccio et al., 2001). As initial preliminary experiments, assessment of brain iron content should therefore be performed in NSE mutants relative to their WT counterparts. This would proceed by harvesting brain tissue for ICP-AES analysis and histological examination using the iron-specific Prussian blue stain, as done previously (Sections 2.3.2 and 2.3.1, respectively).

Owing to differences in the neuronal and cardiac environments, the alterations in gene and protein expression may be different in the brains of NSE mutants compared with the changes that were identified in the hearts of MCK mice (Section 4.3.1). Due to the blood brain barrier, the brain cannot obtain access to the systemic serum iron transport molecule, Tf, and instead, reports indicate that brain neurons possess highly unique pathways by which they metabolise iron (Moos and Morgan, 2004). Examples of brain specific proteins include neuromelanin (Double, 2006, Double et al., 2003, Zecca et al., 2008) neuroglobin (Brunori and Vallone, 2006), and an alternatively spliced, glycosyl phosphatidyl-inositol anchored form of the ferroxidase ceruloplasmin that is only found in the brain (Jeong and David,

2003, Jeong and David, 2006). As an initial screen to identify molecular changes in the NSE brain, laser capture microdissection could be used to isolate neurons from the cerebellum of NSE mutants and their WT littermates according to established protocols (Bitoun et al., 2009, Rossner et al., 2006), after which neurons could be analysed by microarray. Briefly, cerebellum samples would be embedded in O.W.R compound (VWR, West Chester, USA), sectioned at 15 μm using a cryostat microtome, and snap frozen. Sections would then be stained using the LCM Staining Kit Reagent (Ambion, Austin, USA), the neuron-specific antibody, NeuN (Chemicon, Temecula, USA), to identify neurons and Acridine orange (Amresco) and Cresyl violet (Sigma-Aldrich) to visualise RNA and cell morphology, respectively. Laser capture microdissection could then proceed using a Pix-Cell II instrument and Pix-Cell II image archiving workstation (Arturus Engineering, Mountain View, USA). RNA from neurons would then be extracted using an RNAqeous-Micro Kit (Ambion), and first-strand cDNA synthesis and biotin-labeled cRNA performed and hybridized to mouse Affymetrix GeneChips following standard procedures (Dunn et al., 2006, Huang et al., 2009, Thomas and Jankovic, 2004).

In a neural cell line, PIH showed high iron chelation efficacy (Becker and Richardson, 1999), and given the ability of PIH/DFO to prevent iron-loading and alleviate cardiac hypertrophy in the MCK model (Section 4.3.4) (Whitnall et al., 2008), it would be ideal to examine the *in vivo* effect of PIH/DFO on neurodegeneration using the NSE model. However, the aggressive nature of the NSE mutant phenotype (NSE mutant life expectancy is 24 ± 9 days compared with 76 ± 10 days in the MCK mutant) (Puccio et al., 2001) may preclude the use of the PIH/DFO combination for a number of reasons. First, the large molecular size (M_r 657) (Bergeron et al., 1998) and hydrophilic nature of DFO (Aouad et al., 2002) limit its ability to permeate the blood brain barrier (Deloncle et al., 1990), and PIH alone may not be efficient enough to cause significant benefit to this severe model (Whitnall et al., 2008). Previous studies have administered DFO intra-cranially to treat neurodegeneration and neurotoxicity in mouse models of Parkinson's disease (Ben-Shachar et al., 1991, Lan and Jiang, 1997). However in a clinical setting, intracranial injections are not a convenient or practical route of administration. Second, NSE mice are neonatal, and iron deprivation would clearly be detrimental to their already retarded development. Hence, for the study of iron chelation therapy in FA neurodegeneration, a more suitable model would be needed.

6.3.4.2 Other Mouse Models of Friedreich's Ataxia

While other models of neuronal specificity exist (*i.e.*, neuronal changes without cardiac involvement) for the study of FA neuropathology, they do not develop phenotypes associated with FA iron accumulation and are therefore not suitable for examining iron chelation therapy in this disease (Clark et al., 2007, Simon et al., 2004). Alternatively, a number of less aggressive murine models that have both neuronal and cardiac frataxin deficiency exist (Puccio, 2009) and potentially, one of these models could be used to assess the effects of PIH on FA neurodegeneration.

A close reproduction of the human disease is seen in the GAA repeat expansion model (Al-Mahdawi et al., 2006). GAA repeat expansion mutants express reduced levels of frataxin, exhibit markers of oxidative stress and develop both neurodegeneration and cardiac pathology (Al-Mahdawi et al., 2006). Disease progression in the GAA repeat expansion model is extremely slow. Cardiac iron accumulation and significant changes in the phenotype do not develop until mice are > 1 year of age (Al-

185

Mahdawi et al., 2006). This slow pathological development and accumulation of iron may enable the use of PIH alone, in contrast to the more aggressive PIH/DFO combination that was needed to treat the rapid and aggressive phenotype observed in the MCK mutant (as discussed in Section 4.4). However, the delayed development of the phenotype in the GAA repeat expansion model is a considerable practical problem in the research environment, particularly in the initial stages of therapeutic testing. While other murine models of FA do exist, they are not suitable for *in vivo* examination because they are either embryonically lethal (Cossee et al., 2000) or do not develop significant phenotypes suited for the study of chelation in FA (Clark et al., 2007, Miranda et al., 2002, Rai et al., 2008, Ristow et al., 2003, Simon et al., 2004).

6.4 CONDITIONAL FRATAXIN KNOCKOUT IN THE FRIEDREICH'S ATAXIA HEART: TREATMENT BY IRON SUPPLEMENTATION AND DEMONSTRATION OF THE CARDIAC CONTROL OF SYSTEMIC IRON METABOLISM

6.4.1 Significance and Summary of Principal Findings – Chapter 5

The studies performed in Chapter 4 identified the existence of a significant cytosolic iron deficiency in the MCK mutant heart in addition to mitochondrial iron accumulation (Chapter 4) (Whitnall et al., 2008). Both iron deficiency and iron accumulation probably play roles in the pathogenesis of disease (Hentze et al., 2010, Kakhlon et al., 2010). Given this, therapeutic interventions in the MCK mouse, should address iron dysmetabolism that occurs both in the cytosolic and mitochondrial compartment. With this in mind, studies in Chapter 5 were designed to correct the cytosolic iron deficiency by dietary iron supplementation. As a result of these experiments, some important findings were made regarding systemic iron metabolism in the MCK mutant.

Dietary iron significantly ($p < 0.001$) decreased the extent of cardiac hypertrophy in the high iron diet fed mutant, compared to the normal iron diet fed mutant (Figure 5.1B). However, the mechanisms that facilitated this effect were unclear. Possible underlying reasons were discussed in Section 5.4 and hence the reader is referred to this latter section.

Interestingly, frataxin deficiency in mutants, led to the loss of the normal physiologic response to dietary iron loading that was observed in the high iron diet fed WT mice. Despite a slight, but significant ($p < 0.05$) increase

187

in cardiac iron concentration in the high iron diet fed mutant, no change was observed in the expression of the cytosolic iron metabolism proteins, TfR1, H-ferritin and IRP2, or in the ISC-containing proteins SDHA and Fech in the heart (Figure 5.2). This was despite the fact that in WT animals, normal regulation of TfR1 and H-ferritin were observed upon iron loading (Figure 5.2) (Robb and Wessling-Resnick, 2004), *i.e.,* decreased TfR1 and increased H-ferritin expression. This indicates that the normal regulation of iron metabolism in response to increased iron levels is disturbed in the frataxin mutant.

An intriguing and important outcome of the dietary iron loading investigations, was the marked increase in iron concentration that was observed in the liver, spleen and kidney of normal iron diet fed mutants (Figure 5.1D-F). Unlike the frataxin-deficient MCK mutant heart, the liver, spleen and kidney of MCK mutant do express frataxin (Huang et al., 2009, Puccio et al., 2001). Importantly, these results indicate that frataxin deletion in the heart affects systemic iron uptake. Furthermore, they also highlight the significant influence of the heart on systemic iron metabolism. Indeed, interesting changes were observed in the expression of the systemic iron regulatory protein, Hjv, in the heart and the liver (Figure 5.2). This may indicate a possible means by which these two organs can communicate. However, more studies are required to investigate this hypothesis and to examine the systemic iron signalling pathways that are involved.

Given the central role of iron in the pathogenesis of FA, it is surprising that the form of iron accumulating in the FA mitochondrion has not yet been correctly identified. Electron microscopy and measurements of magnetic susceptibility performed in Chapter 5, confirmed that iron does not accumulate in ferritin in the MCK mutant heart. This directly supports the molecular down-regulation of H- and L-ferritin expression detected in Chapter 4. Size-exclusion chromatography, magnetic measurements and the physical appearance of aggregates in transmission electron micrographs indicated that mitochondrial iron in the MCK mutant heart was accumulating as a highly crystalline inorganic compound distinct from the isolated spheres of ferritin that were identified from the liver of these mice (Figure 5.5).

6.4.2 Future Studies Examining Iron Supplementation Therapy

6.4.2.1 Iron Supplementation Using SIH-Fe

A different approach to iron supplementation could involve the lipophilic iron complex of salicylaldehyde isonicotinoyl hydrazone (SIH-Fe). In rapidly replicating reticulocytes, SIH-Fe is able to donate iron to haem metabolic pathways and increase haem synthesis (Laskey et al., 1986, Ponka and Schulman, 1985). Hence, it appears that this low M_r and highly lipophilic iron complex can provide iron to the mitochondrial iron processing machinery. Considering this, SIH-Fe complexes may also be able to donate iron to ISC and haem synthetic pathways that are markedly perturbed in FA (Huang et al., 2009). Indeed, preliminary studies using a tetracycline-inducible model that causes both frataxin and ISC-protein deficiency (as a result of MIT ferritin hyper-expression) (Nie et al., 2005), showed that SIH-Fe can increase the expression of both SDHA and Fech (Figure 6.3) (Austin C and Richardson DR, unpublished data). Future studies should now begin to assess the ability of SIH-Fe to replenish ISC synthesis in the MCK mutant model of FA.

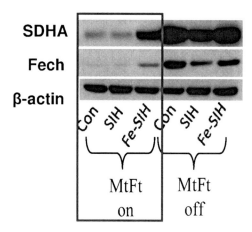

Figure 6.3 SIH-Fe significantly (p < 0.001) increases SDHA and Fech expression in cells that hyper-express MIT ferritin ('MtFt on') as a mechanism to induce frataxin and ISC deficiency (blue box). Printed with permission of C. Austin and D.R. Richardson.

6.4.3 Identifying the Cause of Systemic Iron Overload in the MCK Mouse

Further studies are required to elucidate the mechanisms and pathways that are involved in producing the systemic iron overload (Chapter 5) that occurs following deletion of frataxin from the heart of the MCK mutant (Figures 4.1 and 5.2) (Puccio et al., 2001). Since its discovery in 2001 (Park et al., 2001), the liver-derived hormone, hepcidin, and the liver itself (and associated reticuloendothelial system), have been the focal points of systemic iron research (Hentze et al., 2010, Nemeth, 2010, Pietrangelo, 2010). However, as an iron and energy consuming organ that is crucial for the viability of the circulatory system and thus the organism, it is logical that the heart should also play a vital role in the regulation of systemic iron metabolism. Certainly, studies are beginning to highlight the need to examine the role of the heart, in addition to that of the liver, in the regulation of systemic iron homeostasis (Merle et al., 2007). Interestingly, a mouse model that causes cardiac-specific deletion of the copper metabolism molecule, Ctr1, has recently been generated (Kim et al., 2010). Following deletion of Ctr1 in the heart only, Ctr1 mutant mice develop a phenotype marked by copper deficiency and cardiac hypertrophy (Kim et al., 2010), that is similar to the cytosolic iron deficiency and cardiac hypertrophy observed after frataxin deletion in the MCK mutant (Whitnall et al., 2008). In the context of the present discussion, investigators importantly identified a systemic copper homeostasis regulatory mechanism that is able to signal the copper status of the heart, to tissues involved in copper uptake and storage (such as the liver) (Kim et al., 2010).

While evidence indicates that hepcidin *is* a central regulator of systemic iron (Darshan and Anderson, 2009), less is known of the proteins that in turn influence hepcidin synthesis, such as Hjv and TfR2 (Hentze et al., 2010). Indeed, a complete mechanism of systemic iron regulation has not yet been comprehensively elucidated.

Many mechanisms involved in iron metabolism have been deciphered through the analysis of disease or mutant animals (Huang et al., 2009), such as the mutations in the Hjv-encoding gene *HFE2* in juvenile haemochromatosis, that first identified the critical involvement of Hjv in iron metabolism (Papanikolaou et al., 2004). In fact what might be discovered, is that studies using the MCK mutant model could be the first to demonstrate the precise signalling cascades that underlie systemic communication between organs such as the heart and the liver.

6.4.3.1 Hepcidin and Ferroportin1

Given that ferroportin1 in duodenal enterocytes is the "gateway" of external iron absorption into the body (Donovan et al., 2005), western blotting (Section 2.5) could be performed on duodenal tissue from MCK mutants and WT mice using the ferroportin1 antibody from Section 4.2.5. Both 4- and 9-week old MCK mutant and WT mice could be examined, to identify changes in protein expression over time. Considering the increased iron loading of the liver, spleen and kidney, we may expect that ferroportin1 may be up-regulated, leading to increased iron uptake from the gut in MCK mutant relative to WT mice.

Considering hepcidin is a principal regulator of dietary iron absorption *via* its affect on ferroportin1 in duodenal enterocytes (Nemeth et al., 2004), and that hepcidin is chiefly synthesised in the liver, western blotting on 4- and 9-week old MCK mutant and WT liver could be performed. To do this, a commercially available antibody that recognises the active 25 amino acid hepcidin peptide could be used (Sigma-Aldrich). In addition to the liver, hepcidin is also expressed in the heart, albeit at a much lower level (Merle et al., 2007), and thus, western blotting could also be performed on this organ. This may help to elucidate if the heart uses hepcidin directly as a method of manipulating ferroportin1 on duodenal enterocytes.

Ideally, it would also be desirable to quantitate levels of circulating hepcidin-25 in the serum of MCK mutant compared to WT mice. A number of methods have recently been developed to assess hepcidin, including surface-enhanced laser desorption/ionization- and matrix assisted laser desorption/ionization-time-of-flight mass spectrometry (*i.e.,* SELDI-TOF MS and MALDI-TOF MS, respectively) (Bozzini et al., 2008, Swinkels et al., 2008, Ward et al., 2008), liquid chromatography tandem-MS (*i.e.,* LC-MS/MS) (Bansal et al., 2009, Murao et al., 2007), radioimmunoassays (RIAs) (Ashby et al., 2009, Busbridge et al., 2009, Grebenchtchikov et al., 2009) and enzyme-linked immunosorbent assays (ELISAs) (Ganz et al.,

2008, Koliaraki et al., 2009). However, at this stage, there is no universal technique for measuring hepcidin in the blood, and significant variations have been found between methods (Kroot et al., 2009). These inter-method differences may arise due to variations in calibration and antibodies that are used in each method (Kroot et al., 2009). Furthermore, detection of hepcidin could be masked by circulating serum proteins such as albumin, immunoglobulin G (Brasse-Lagnel et al., 2010, Schwarz et al., 2010), and particularly α_2-macroglobulin, that binds specifically to hepcidin in the plasma (Peslova et al., 2009). Hence, any estimation of circulating hepcidin must take these factors into account. Currently, work is underway to 'harmonise' the various hepcidin assays by introducing internal standards and methods for calibration (Kroot et al., 2009). Perhaps when these problems have been resolved, an ELISA or RIA may be available to enable precise and accurate quantitation of hepcidin in the serum of MCK mice.

6.4.3.2 Protein Regulators of Hepcidin Expression

An array of systemic stimuli regulate hepcidin synthesis (Darshan and Anderson, 2009, Hentze et al., 2010). Significant differences were observed in the expression of the hepcidin-regulatory molecule (Zhang et al., 2010), Hjv, between MCK mutant and WT mice within the heart and the liver (Figure 5.2). Considering this, future studies could involve an examination of the hepatocyte cell surface proteins, TfR2 and HFE, that in conjunction to Hjv, activate the BMP-SMAD signal transduction pathway to regulate hepcidin expression in the hepatocyte (Darshan and Anderson, 2009). Indeed, mutations in hepcidin and in the genes that code for Hjv, TfR2 and HFE, cause severe forms of hereditary haemochromatosis (Camaschella, 2005). Additionally, the form of Hjv detected in Chapter 5 (*i.e.,* sHjv or mHjv), must be clarified. Gene array and RT-PCR studies demonstrate that a reasonable level of *Hfe2* mRNA (that encodes Hjv) is expressed in the MCK mutant heart (Huang et al., 2009). However, Hjv protein expression was negligible in the MCK mutant heart (Figure 5.2A). This indicates that post-translational events may be responsible for the changes in Hjv protein expression. For example, cleavage of Hjv may occur by the proprotein convertase, furin, which releases Hjv from cells to generate sHjv (Silvestri et al., 2008). Expression of *Furin* mRNA is mediated by iron and hypoxia (Poli et al., 2010, Silvestri et al., 2008), and western blotting of MCK mutant and WT heart tissue could be examined using the commercially available anti-furin antibody from Santa Cruz Biotechnology (Santa Cruz, USA). Up-regulation of furin after western blotting may therefore indicate there is increased cleavage of Hjv to the sHjv form, and thus, increased generation of sHjv. If sHjv is quickly secreted into the serum, it may prevent the detection of sHjv in the tissue, and thus it would be important to investigate sHjv expression in the serum (Silvestri et al., 2008). Methods for examining Hjv expression in the serum are currently being established (Brasse-Lagnel et al., 2010).

In hepatocytes, HFE has been suggested to act as a bimodal switch between TfR1 and TfR2 on the plasma membrane (Goswami and Andrews, 2006). Hepcidin activation by holo-transferrin involves both HFE and TfR2 (Gao et al., 2010). The Tfr1-HFE-TfR2 relationship is only just beginning to be elucidated. A current model suggests that high serum Tf-Fe concentrations displace HFE from TfR1, to promote its interaction with TfR2 (Hentze et al., 2010). Considering this, western blotting (Section 2.5) could be performed on MCK mutant and WT liver tissue, using TfR2 and HFE antibodies from Santa Cruz Biotechnology (Santa Cruz, USA). Results may also help explain the changes that were observed in TfR1 expression in the MCK mutant liver in Chapter 5 (Figure 5.2B).

6.4.4 Identifying the Form of Iron in the Mitochondrion of the MCK Mouse

Identifying the form of iron accumulating in the FA mitochondrion may lead to the generation of better pharmaceutical agents for the treatment of this disease. It may also result in a better understanding of the function of frataxin and its interactions with iron. Indeed, during mythe current studies, a number of techniques were tested in an attempt to characterise the form of iron that accumulates in the MCK mutant heart. Trialled techniques included: (i) electron paramagnetic resonance spectroscopy; (ii) near-infrared Raman spectroscopy; (iii) Mössbauer spectroscopy; and (iv) X-ray absorption near edge spectroscopy. However, for each of these techniques, significant problems, such as poor signal-to-noise ratio, were encountered, and little useful information was obtained from these investigations.

To complement the ultrastructural analysis of TEM sections in Section 5.3.4.2, selected area surface diffraction could be performed, using a JEOL 1200 EXII TEM (Peabody, USA) operated at 100 kV (Gutiérrez et al., 2006) to examine the MCK mutant heart and liver sections prepared in Section 5.2.5. The use of concomitant electron microscopy with this technique, would allow electron microdiffraction patterns of the electron-dense mitochondrial iron aggregates to be directly collected. Diffraction patterns of the iron aggregates could be compared to patterns of already identified material such as ferrihydrite, haematite and goethite (Gutiérrez et al., 2006, Gutiérrez et al., 2009), and hence, this technique may more closely indicate the nature and form of iron in the MCK mutant mitochondrion.

6.5 CONCLUDING REMARKS

In summary, the data presented within this thesis demonstrates how iron chelators can be employed for the treatment of cancer (Whitnall et al., 2006) and FA (Whitnall et al., 2008, Whitnall and Richardson, 2006). Moreover, the work also demonstrates the marked changes in iron metabolism that occur at a cellular (Whitnall et al., 2008) and systemic level in FA. The future studies suggested above could potentially lead to the clinical use of Dp44mT or Dp44mT-like chelators for the treatment of cancer. They could also lead to the development of appropriate iron chelators and iron complexes to address the iron accumulation and ISC- and haem-deficiencies in FA, respectively. Furthermore, future analysis of the MCK model of FA may increase our present knowledge of systemic iron metabolism in general, and raise awareness of the role of the heart in regulating iron processing.

CHAPTER 7
REFERENCES

ABDELAZIZ, A. I., PAGEL, I., SCHLEGEL, W. P., KOTT, M., MONTI, J., HAASE, H. & MORANO, I. (2005) Human atrial myosin light chain 1 expression attenuates heart failure. *Adv Exp Med Biol,* 565, 283-92; discussion 92, 405-15.

ABEYSINGHE, R. D., GREENE, B. T., HAYNES, R., WILLINGHAM, M. C., TURNER, J., PLANALP, R. P., BRECHBIEL, M. W., TORTI, F. M. & TORTI, S. V. (2001) p53-independent apoptosis mediated by tachpyridine, an anti-cancer iron chelator. *Carcinogenesis,* 22, 1607-14.

AISEN, P., LEIBMAN, A. & ZWEIER, J. (1978) Stoichiometric and site characteristics of the binding of iron to human transferrin. *J Biol Chem,* 253, 1930-7.

AJIOKA, R. S., PHILLIPS, J. D. & KUSHNER, J. P. (2006) Biosynthesis of heme in mammals. *Biochim Biophys Acta,* 1763, 723-36.

AKIYAMA, S., FOJO, A., HANOVER, J. A., PASTAN, I. & GOTTESMAN, M. M. (1985) Isolation and genetic characterization of human KB cell lines resistant to multiple drugs. *Somat Cell Mol Genet,* 11, 117-26.

AL-MAHDAWI, S., PINTO, R. M., VARSHNEY, D., LAWRENCE, L., LOWRIE, M. B., HUGHES, S., WEBSTER, Z., BLAKE, J., COOPER, J. M., KING, R. & POOK, M. A. (2006) GAA repeat expansion mutation mouse models of Friedreich ataxia exhibit oxidative stress leading to progressive neuronal and cardiac pathology. *Genomics,* 88, 580-90.

ALLEMANN, E., GURNY, R., DOELKER, E., SKINNER, F. S. & SCHEUETZ, H. (1994) Distribution kinetics and elimination of radioactivity after intravenous intramuscular injection of 14C-savoxepine loaded poly(DL-lactic acid) nanospheres to rats. *J Control Release,* 29, 97-104.

ALLEN, P. D., ST PIERRE, T. G., CHUA-ANUSORN, W., STROM, V. & RAO, K. V. (2000) Low-frequency low-field magnetic susceptibility of ferritin and hemosiderin. *Biochim Biophys Acta,* 1500, 186-96.

ALLIKMETS, R., RASKIND, W. H., HUTCHINSON, A., SCHUECK, N. D., DEAN, M. & KOELLER, D. M. (1999) Mutation of a putative mitochondrial iron transporter gene (ABC7) in X-linked sideroblastic anemia and ataxia (XLSA/A). *Hum Mol Genet,* 8, 743-9.

ALPER, G. & NARAYANAN, V. (2003) Friedreich's ataxia. *Pediatr Neurol,* 28, 335-41.

ANDERSON, G. J. & VULPE, C. D. (2009) Mammalian iron transport. *Cell Mol Life Sci,* 66, 3241-61.

AOUAD, F., FLORENCE, A., ZHANG, Y., COLLINS, F., HENRY, C., WARD, R. J. & CHRICTON, R. R. (2002) Evaluation of new iron chelators and their therapeutic potential. *Inorg. Chim. Acta,* 339, 470-480.

AOUALI, N., EDDABRA, L., MACADRE, J. & MORJANI, H. (2005) Immunosuppressors and reversion of multidrug-resistance. *Crit Rev Oncol Hematol,* 56, 61-70.

AROSIO, P., ADELMAN, T. G. & DRYSDALE, J. W. (1978) On ferritin heterogeneity. Further evidence for heteropolymers. *J Biol Chem,* 253, 4451-8.

AROSIO, P., INGRASSIA, R. & CAVADINI, P. (2009) Ferritins: a family of molecules for iron storage, antioxidation and more. *Biochim Biophys Acta,* 1790, 589-99.

ASHBY, D. R., GALE, D. P., BUSBRIDGE, M., MURPHY, K. G., DUNCAN, N. D., CAIRNS, T. D., TAUBE, D. H., BLOOM, S. R., TAM, F. W., CHAPMAN, R. S., MAXWELL, P. H. & CHOI, P. (2009) Plasma hepcidin levels are elevated but responsive to erythropoietin therapy in renal disease. *Kidney Int,* 75, 976-81.

ATWOOD, C. S., HUANG, X., MOIR, R. D., TANZI, R. E. & BUSH, A. I. (1999) Role of free radicals and metal ions in the pathogenesis of Alzheimer's disease. *Met Ions Biol Syst,* 36, 309-64.

BABCOCK, M., DE SILVA, D., OAKS, R., DAVIS-KAPLAN, S., JIRALERSPONG, S., MONTERMINI, L., PANDOLFO, M. & KAPLAN, J. (1997) Regulation of mitochondrial iron accumulation by Yfh1p, a putative homolog of frataxin. *Science,* 276, 1709-12.

BABITT, J. L., HUANG, F. W., XIA, Y., SIDIS, Y., ANDREWS, N. C. & LIN, H. Y. (2007) Modulation of bone morphogenetic protein signaling in vivo regulates systemic iron balance. *J Clin Invest,* 117, 1933-9.

BABUSIAK, M., MAN, P., SUTAK, R., PETRAK, J. & VYORAL, D. (2005) Identification of heme binding protein complexes in murine erythroleukemic cells: study by a novel two-dimensional native separation -- liquid chromatography and electrophoresis. *Proteomics,* 5, 340-50.

BALSARI, A., TORTORETO, M., BESUSSO, D., PETRANGOLINI, G., SFONDRINI, L., MAGGI, R., MENARD, S. & PRATESI, G. (2004) Combination of a CpG-oligodeoxynucleotide and a topoisomerase I inhibitor in the therapy of human tumour xenografts. *Eur J Cancer,* 40, 1275-81.

BANDYOPADHYAY, S., PAI, S. K., GROSS, S. C., HIROTA, S., HOSOBE, S., MIURA, K., SAITO, K., COMMES, T., HAYASHI, S.,

WATABE, M. & WATABE, K. (2003) The Drg-1 gene suppresses tumor metastasis in prostate cancer. *Cancer Res,* 63, 1731-6.

BANDYOPADHYAY, S., PAI, S. K., HIROTA, S., HOSOBE, S., TAKANO, Y., SAITO, K., PIQUEMAL, D., COMMES, T., WATABE, M., GROSS, S. C., WANG, Y., RAN, S. & WATABE, K. (2004a) Role of the putative tumor metastasis suppressor gene Drg-1 in breast cancer progression. *Oncogene,* 23, 5675-81.

BANDYOPADHYAY, S., PAI, S. K., HIROTA, S., HOSOBE, S., TSUKADA, T., MIURA, K., TAKANO, Y., SAITO, K., COMMES, T., PIQUEMAL, D., WATABE, M., GROSS, S., WANG, Y., HUGGENVIK, J. & WATABE, K. (2004b) PTEN up-regulates the tumor metastasis suppressor gene Drg-1 in prostate and breast cancer. *Cancer Res,* 64, 7655-60.

BANSAL, S. S., HALKET, J. M., BOMFORD, A., SIMPSON, R. J., VASAVDA, N., THEIN, S. L. & HIDER, R. C. (2009) Quantitation of hepcidin in human urine by liquid chromatography-mass spectrometry. *Anal Biochem,* 384, 245-53.

BARBEITO, A. G., LEVADE, T., DELISLE, M. B., GHETTI, B. & VIDAL, R. (2010) Abnormal iron metabolism in fibroblasts from a patient with the neurodegenerative disease hereditary ferritinopathy. *Mol Neurodegener,* 5, 50.

BARNHAM, K. J., MASTERS, C. L. & BUSH, A. I. (2004) Neurodegenerative diseases and oxidative stress. *Nat Rev Drug Discov,* 3, 205-14.

BARTZOKIS, G., BECKSON, M., HANCE, D. B., MARX, P., FOSTER, J. A. & MARDER, S. R. (1997) MR evaluation of age-related increase of brain iron in young adults and older normal males. *Magn Reson Imaging*, 15, 29-35.

BECKER, E. & RICHARDSON, D. R. (1999) Development of novel aroylhydrazone ligands for iron chelation therapy: 2-pyridylcarboxaldehyde isonicotinoyl hydrazone analogs. *J Lab Clin Med*, 134, 510-21.

BECKER, E. M., LOVEJOY, D. B., GREER, J. M., WATTS, R. & RICHARDSON, D. R. (2003) Identification of the di-pyridyl ketone isonicotinoyl hydrazone (PKIH) analogues as potent iron chelators and anti-tumour agents. *Br J Pharmacol*, 138, 819-30.

BEKRI, S., KISPAL, G., LANGE, H., FITZSIMONS, E., TOLMIE, J., LILL, R. & BISHOP, D. F. (2000) Human ABC7 transporter: gene structure and mutation causing X-linked sideroblastic anemia with ataxia with disruption of cytosolic iron-sulfur protein maturation. *Blood*, 96, 3256-64.

BEN-SHACHAR, D., ESHEL, G., FINBERG, J. P. & YOUDIM, M. B. (1991) The iron chelator desferrioxamine (Desferal) retards 6-hydroxydopamine-induced degeneration of nigrostriatal dopamine neurons. *J Neurochem*, 56, 1441-4.

BENDOVA, P., MACKOVA, E., HASKOVA, P., VAVROVA, A., JIRKOVSKY, E., STERBA, M., POPELOVA, O., KALINOWSKI, D. S., KOVARIKOVA, P., VAVROVA, K., RICHARDSON, D. R. & SIMUNEK, T. (2010) Comparison of clinically used and experimental iron chelators for protection against oxidative stress-induced cellular injury. *Chem Res Toxicol*, 23, 1105-14.

BERGERON, R. J., WIEGAND, J. & BRITTENHAM, G. M. (1998) HBED: A potential alternative to deferoxamine for iron-chelating therapy. *Blood,* 91, 1446-52.

BERNHARDT, P. V., CALDWELL, L. M., CHASTON, T. B., CHIN, P. & RICHARDSON, D. R. (2003) Cytotoxic iron chelators: characterization of the structure, solution chemistry and redox activity of ligands and iron complexes of the di-2-pyridyl ketone isonicotinoyl hydrazone (HPKIH) analogues. *J Biol Inorg Chem,* 8, 866-80.

BEUTLER, E., GELBART, T., LEE, P., TREVINO, R., FERNANDEZ, M. A. & FAIRBANKS, V. F. (2000) Molecular characterization of a case of atransferrinemia. *Blood,* 96, 4071-4.

BITOUN, E., FINELLI, M. J., OLIVER, P. L., LEE, S. & DAVIES, K. E. (2009) AF4 is a critical regulator of the IGF-1 signaling pathway during Purkinje cell development. *J Neurosci,* 29, 15366-74.

BLATT, J. & STITELY, S. (1987) Antineuroblastoma activity of desferoxamine in human cell lines. *Cancer Res,* 47, 1749-50.

BODDAERT, N., LE QUAN SANG, K. H., ROTIG, A., LEROY-WILLIG, A., GALLET, S., BRUNELLE, F., SIDI, D., THALABARD, J. C., MUNNICH, A. & CABANTCHIK, Z. I. (2007) Selective iron chelation in Friedreich ataxia: biologic and clinical implications. *Blood,* 110, 401-8.

BOZZINI, C., CAMPOSTRINI, N., TROMBINI, P., NEMETH, E., CASTAGNA, A., TENUTI, I., CORROCHER, R., CAMASCHELLA, C., GANZ, T., OLIVIERI, O., PIPERNO, A. & GIRELLI, D. (2008) Measurement of urinary hepcidin levels by SELDI-TOF-MS in HFE-hemochromatosis. *Blood Cells Mol Dis,* 40, 347-52.

BRADLEY, J. L., BLAKE, J. C., CHAMBERLAIN, S., THOMAS, P. K., COOPER, J. M. & SCHAPIRA, A. H. (2000) Clinical, biochemical and molecular genetic correlations in Friedreich's ataxia. *Hum Mol Genet,* 9, 275-82.

BRADLEY, J. L., HOMAYOUN, S., HART, P. E., SCHAPIRA, A. H. & COOPER, J. M. (2004) Role of oxidative damage in Friedreich's ataxia. *Neurochem Res,* 29, 561-7.

BRASSE-LAGNEL, C. G., POLI, M., LESUEUR, C., GRANDCHAMP, B., LAVOINNE, A., BEAUMONT, C. & BEKRI, S. (2010) Immunoassay for human serum hemojuvelin. *Haematologica.*

BRITTENHAM, G. M. (1990) Pyridoxal isonicotinoyl hydrazone: an effective iron-chelator after oral administration. *Semin Hematol,* 27, 112-6.

BRODIE, C., SIRIWARDANA, G., LUCAS, J., SCHLEICHER, R., TERADA, N., SZEPESI, A., GELFAND, E. & SELIGMAN, P. (1993) Neuroblastoma sensitivity to growth inhibition by deferrioxamine: evidence for a block in G1 phase of the cell cycle. *Cancer Res,* 53, 3968-75.

BRUNORI, M. & VALLONE, B. (2006) A globin for the brain. *FASEB J,* 20, 2192-7.

BURDO, J. R. & CONNOR, J. R. (2003) Brain iron uptake and homeostatic mechanisms: an overview. *Biometals,* 16, 63-75.

BUSBRIDGE, M., GRIFFITHS, C., ASHBY, D., GALE, D., JAYANTHA, A., SANWAIYA, A. & CHAPMAN, R. S. (2009) Development of a novel immunoassay for the iron regulatory peptide hepcidin. *Br J Biomed Sci,* 66, 150-7.

BUSH, A. I. & TANZI, R. E. (2002) The galvanization of beta-amyloid in Alzheimer's disease. *Proc Natl Acad Sci U S A,* 99, 7317-9.

BUSS, J. L., GREENE, B. T., TURNER, J., TORTI, F. M. & TORTI, S. V. (2004) Iron chelators in cancer chemotherapy. *Curr Top Med Chem,* 4, 1623-35.

CABANTCHIK, Z. I., BREUER, W., ZANNINELLI, G. & CIANCIULLI, P. (2005) LPI-labile plasma iron in iron overload. *Best Pract Res Clin Haematol,* 18, 277-87.

CALABRESE, V., LODI, R., TONON, C., D'AGATA, V., SAPIENZA, M., SCAPAGNINI, G., MANGIAMELI, A., PENNISI, G., STELLA, A. M. & BUTTERFIELD, D. A. (2005) Oxidative stress, mitochondrial dysfunction and cellular stress response in Friedreich's ataxia. *J Neurol Sci,* 233, 145-62.

CAMASCHELLA, C. (2005) Understanding iron homeostasis through genetic analysis of hemochromatosis and related disorders. *Blood,* 106, 3710-7.

CAMPANELLA, A., ISAYA, G., O'NEILL, H. A., SANTAMBROGIO, P., COZZI, A., AROSIO, P. & LEVI, S. (2004) The expression of human mitochondrial ferritin rescues respiratory function in frataxin-deficient yeast. *Hum Mol Genet,* 13, 2279-88.

CAMPANELLA, A., ROVELLI, E., SANTAMBROGIO, P., COZZI, A., TARONI, F. & LEVI, S. (2009) Mitochondrial ferritin limits oxidative damage regulating mitochondrial iron availability: hypothesis for a protective role in Friedreich ataxia. *Hum Mol Genet,* 18, 1-11.

CAMPUZANO, V., MONTERMINI, L., LUTZ, Y., COVA, L., HINDELANG, C., JIRALERSPONG, S., TROTTIER, Y., KISH, S. J., FAUCHEUX, B., TROUILLAS, P., AUTHIER, F. J., DURR, A., MANDEL, J. L., VESCOVI, A., PANDOLFO, M. & KOENIG, M. (1997) Frataxin is reduced in Friedreich ataxia patients and is associated with mitochondrial membranes. *Hum Mol Genet,* 6, 1771-80.

CAMPUZANO, V., MONTERMINI, L., MOLTO, M. D., PIANESE, L., COSSEE, M., CAVALCANTI, F., MONROS, E., RODIUS, F., DUCLOS, F., MONTICELLI, A., ZARA, F., CANIZARES, J., KOUTNIKOVA, H., BIDICHANDANI, S. I., GELLERA, C., BRICE, A., TROUILLAS, P., DE MICHELE, G., FILLA, A., DE FRUTOS, R., PALAU, F., PATEL, P. I., DI DONATO, S., MANDEL, J. L., COCOZZA, S., KOENIG, M. & PANDOLFO, M. (1996) Friedreich's ataxia: autosomal recessive disease caused by an intronic GAA triplet repeat expansion. *Science,* 271, 1423-7.

CARRETERO, J., MEDINA, P. P., PIO, R., MONTUENGA, L. M. & SANCHEZ-CESPEDES, M. (2004) Novel and natural knockout lung cancer cell lines for the LKB1/STK11 tumor suppressor gene. *Oncogene,* 23, 4037-40.

CAVADINI, P., BIASIOTTO, G., POLI, M., LEVI, S., VERARDI, R., ZANELLA, I., DEROSAS, M., INGRASSIA, R., CORRADO, M. & AROSIO, P. (2007) RNA silencing of the mitochondrial ABCB7 transporter in HeLa cells causes an iron-deficient phenotype with mitochondrial iron overload. *Blood,* 109, 3552-9.

CHANDEL, N. S., MCCLINTOCK, D. S., FELICIANO, C. E., WOOD, T. M., MELENDEZ, J. A., RODRIGUEZ, A. M. & SCHUMACKER, P. T. (2000) Reactive oxygen species generated at mitochondrial complex III stabilize hypoxia-inducible factor-1alpha during hypoxia: a mechanism of O2 sensing. *J Biol Chem,* 275, 25130-8.

CHASTEEN, N. D. & HARRISON, P. M. (1999) Mineralization in ferritin: an efficient means of iron storage. *J Struct Biol,* 126, 182-94.

CHASTON, T. B., LOVEJOY, D. B., WATTS, R. N. & RICHARDSON, D. R. (2003) Examination of the antiproliferative activity of iron chelators: multiple cellular targets and the different mechanism of action of triapine compared with desferrioxamine and the potent pyridoxal isonicotinoyl hydrazone analogue 311. *Clin Cancer Res,* 9, 402-14.

CHASTON, T. B. & RICHARDSON, D. R. (2003a) Interactions of the pyridine-2-carboxaldehyde isonicotinoyl hydrazone class of chelators with iron and DNA: implications for toxicity in the treatment of iron overload disease. *J Biol Inorg Chem,* 8, 427-38.

CHASTON, T. B. & RICHARDSON, D. R. (2003b) Iron chelators for the treatment of iron overload disease: relationship between structure, redox activity, and toxicity. *Am J Hematol,* 73, 200-10.

CHASTON, T. B., WATTS, R. N., YUAN, J. & RICHARDSON, D. R. (2004) Potent antitumor activity of novel iron chelators derived from di-2-pyridylketone isonicotinoyl hydrazone involves fenton-derived free radical generation. *Clin Cancer Res,* 10, 7365-74.

CHEN, O. S., HEMENWAY, S. & KAPLAN, J. (2002) Inhibition of Fe-S cluster biosynthesis decreases mitochondrial iron export: evidence that

Yfh1p affects Fe-S cluster synthesis. *Proc Natl Acad Sci U S A,* 99, 12321-6.

CHEN, W., DAILEY, H. A. & PAW, B. H. (2010) Ferrochelatase forms an oligomeric complex with mitoferrin-1 and Abcb10 for erythroid heme biosynthesis. *Blood,* 116, 628-30.

CHEN, W., PARADKAR, P. N., LI, L., PIERCE, E. L., LANGER, N. B., TAKAHASHI-MAKISE, N., HYDE, B. B., SHIRIHAI, O. S., WARD, D. M., KAPLAN, J. & PAW, B. H. (2009) Abcb10 physically interacts with mitoferrin-1 (Slc25a37) to enhance its stability and function in the erythroid mitochondria. *Proc Natl Acad Sci U S A,* 106, 16263-8.

CHI, T. Y., CHEN, G. G. & LAI, P. B. (2004) Eicosapentaenoic acid induces Fas-mediated apoptosis through a p53-dependent pathway in hepatoma cells. *Cancer J,* 10, 190-200.

CHONG, T. W., HORWITZ, L. D., MOORE, J. W., SOWTER, H. M. & HARRIS, A. L. (2002) A mycobacterial iron chelator, desferri-exochelin, induces hypoxia-inducible factors 1 and 2, NIP3, and vascular endothelial growth factor in cancer cell lines. *Cancer Res,* 62, 6924-7.

CHUA, A. C., DELIMA, R. D., MORGAN, E. H., HERBISON, C. E., TIRNITZ-PARKER, J. E., GRAHAM, R. M., FLEMING, R. E., BRITTON, R. S., BACON, B. R., OLYNYK, J. K. & TRINDER, D. (2010) Iron uptake from plasma transferrin by a transferrin receptor 2 mutant mouse model of haemochromatosis. *J Hepatol,* 52, 425-31.

CIKRT, M., PONKA, P., NECAS, E. & NEUWIRT, J. (1980) Biliary iron excretion in rats following pyridoxal isonicotinoyl hydrazone. *Br J Haematol,* 45, 275-83.

CLARK, R. M., DE BIASE, I., MALYKHINA, A. P., AL-MAHDAWI, S., POOK, M. & BIDICHANDANI, S. I. (2007) The GAA triplet-repeat is unstable in the context of the human FXN locus and displays age-dependent expansions in cerebellum and DRG in a transgenic mouse model. *Hum Genet,* 120, 633-40.

COLDHAM, N. G., ZHANG, A. Q., KEY, P. & SAUER, M. J. (2002) Absolute bioavailability of [14C] genistein in the rat; plasma pharmacokinetics of parent compound, genistein glucuronide and total radioactivity. *Eur J Drug Metab Pharmacokinet,* 27, 249-58.

CONNOR, J. R., SNYDER, B. S., BEARD, J. L., FINE, R. E. & MUFSON, E. J. (1992) Regional distribution of iron and iron-regulatory proteins in the brain in aging and Alzheimer's disease. *J Neurosci Res,* 31, 327-35.

COOK, S. D. (2007) Approved drugs and their problems in patient care: routes of administration and dosing. *J Neurol Sci,* 259, 38-41.

COSSEE, M., PUCCIO, H., GANSMULLER, A., KOUTNIKOVA, H., DIERICH, A., LEMEUR, M., FISCHBECK, K., DOLLE, P. & KOENIG, M. (2000) Inactivation of the Friedreich ataxia mouse gene leads to early embryonic lethality without iron accumulation. *Hum Mol Genet,* 9, 1219-26.

CREMONESI, L., FOGLIENI, B., FERMO, I., COZZI, A., PARONI, R., RUGGERI, G., BELLOLI, S., LEVI, S., FARGION, S., FERRARI, M. & AROSIO, P. (2003) Identification of two novel mutations in the 5'-untranslated region of H-ferritin using denaturing high performance liquid chromatography scanning. *Haematologica,* 88, 1110-6.

CRONAUER, M. V., SCHULZ, W. A., BURCHARDT, T., ACKERMANN, R. & BURCHARDT, M. (2004) Inhibition of p53 function diminishes androgen receptor-mediated signaling in prostate cancer cell lines. *Oncogene,* 23, 3541-9.

CUNNINGHAM, M. J. & NATHAN, D. G. (2005) New developments in iron chelators. *Curr Opin Hematol,* 12, 129-34.

CURTIS, A. R., FEY, C., MORRIS, C. M., BINDOFF, L. A., INCE, P. G., CHINNERY, P. F., COULTHARD, A., JACKSON, M. J., JACKSON, A. P., MCHALE, D. P., HAY, D., BARKER, W. A., MARKHAM, A. F., BATES, D., CURTIS, A. & BURN, J. (2001) Mutation in the gene encoding ferritin light polypeptide causes dominant adult-onset basal ganglia disease. *Nat Genet,* 28, 350-4.

DARNELL, G. & RICHARDSON, D. R. (1999) The potential of iron chelators of the pyridoxal isonicotinoyl hydrazone class as effective antiproliferative agents III: the effect of the ligands on molecular targets involved in proliferation. *Blood,* 94, 781-92.

DARSHAN, D. & ANDERSON, G. J. (2009) Interacting signals in the control of hepcidin expression. *Biometals,* 22, 77-87.

DARSHAN, D., VANOAICA, L., RICHMAN, L., BEERMANN, F. & KUHN, L. C. (2009) Conditional deletion of ferritin H in mice induces loss of iron storage and liver damage. *Hepatology,* 50, 852-60.

DE MICHELE, G., PERRONE, F., FILLA, A., MIRANTE, E., GIORDANO, M., DE PLACIDO, S. & CAMPANELLA, G. (1996) Age of onset, sex, and cardiomyopathy as predictors of disability and survival in Friedreich's disease: a retrospective study on 119 patients. *Neurology,* 47, 1260-4.

DELATYCKI, M. B., WILLIAMSON, R. & FORREST, S. M. (2000) Friedreich ataxia: an overview. *J Med Genet,* 37, 1-8.

DELONCLE, R., GUILLARD, O., CLANET, F., COURTOIS, P. & PIRIOU, A. (1990) Aluminum transfer as glutamate complex through blood-brain barrier. Possible implication in dialysis encephalopathy. *Biol Trace Elem Res,* 25, 39-45.

DI PROSPERO, N. A., BAKER, A., JEFFRIES, N. & FISCHBECK, K. H. (2007) Neurological effects of high-dose idebenone in patients with Friedreich's ataxia: a randomised, placebo-controlled trial. *Lancet Neurol,* 6, 878-86.

DONFRANCESCO, A., DEB, G., DOMINICI, C., PILEGGI, D., CASTELLO, M. A. & HELSON, L. (1990) Effects of a single course of deferoxamine in neuroblastoma patients. *Cancer Res,* 50, 4929-30.

DONG, Y. B., YANG, H. L., ELLIOTT, M. J., LIU, T. J., STILWELL, A., ATIENZA, C., JR. & MCMASTERS, K. M. (1999) Adenovirus-mediated E2F-1 gene transfer efficiently induces apoptosis in melanoma cells. *Cancer,* 86, 2021-33.

DONOVAN, A., LIMA, C. A., PINKUS, J. L., PINKUS, G. S., ZON, L. I., ROBINE, S. & ANDREWS, N. C. (2005) The iron exporter ferroportin/Slc40a1 is essential for iron homeostasis. *Cell Metab,* 1, 191-200.

DOUBLE, K. L. (2006) Functional effects of neuromelanin and synthetic melanin in model systems. *J Neural Transm,* 113, 751-6.

DOUBLE, K. L., GERLACH, M., SCHUNEMANN, V., TRAUTWEIN, A. X., ZECCA, L., GALLORINI, M., YOUDIM, M. B., RIEDERER, P.

& BEN-SHACHAR, D. (2003) Iron-binding characteristics of neuromelanin of the human substantia nigra. *Biochem Pharmacol*, 66, 489-94.

DRYSDALE, J. W. & MUNRO, H. N. (1966) Regulation of synthesis and turnover of ferritin in rat liver. *J Biol Chem*, 241, 3630-7.

DUNN, L. L., RAHMANTO, Y. S. & RICHARDSON, D. R. (2007) Iron uptake and metabolism in the new millennium. *Trends Cell Biol*, 17, 93-100.

DUNN, L. L., SEKYERE, E. O., RAHMANTO, Y. S. & RICHARDSON, D. R. (2006) The function of melanotransferrin: a role in melanoma cell proliferation and tumorigenesis. *Carcinogenesis*, 27, 2157-69.

DURR, A., COSSEE, M., AGID, Y., CAMPUZANO, V., MIGNARD, C., PENET, C., MANDEL, J. L., BRICE, A. & KOENIG, M. (1996) Clinical and genetic abnormalities in patients with Friedreich's ataxia. *N Engl J Med*, 335, 1169-75.

EATON, J. W. & QIAN, M. (2002) Molecular bases of cellular iron toxicity. *Free Radic Biol Med*, 32, 833-40.

EL-AGNAF, O. M. & IRVINE, G. B. (2002) Aggregation and neurotoxicity of alpha-synuclein and related peptides. *Biochem Soc Trans*, 30, 559-65.

ESPOSITO, B. P., BREUER, W., SIRANKAPRACHA, P., POOTRAKUL, P., HERSHKO, C. & CABANTCHIK, Z. I. (2003) Labile plasma iron in iron overload: redox activity and susceptibility to chelation. *Blood*, 102, 2670-7.

FAUCHEUX, B. A., MARTIN, M. E., BEAUMONT, C., HAUW, J. J., AGID, Y. & HIRSCH, E. C. (2003) Neuromelanin associated redox-active iron is increased in the substantia nigra of patients with Parkinson's disease. *J Neurochem,* 86, 1142-8.

FAUCHEUX, B. A., MARTIN, M. E., BEAUMONT, C., HUNOT, S., HAUW, J. J., AGID, Y. & HIRSCH, E. C. (2002) Lack of up-regulation of ferritin is associated with sustained iron regulatory protein-1 binding activity in the substantia nigra of patients with Parkinson's disease. *J Neurochem,* 83, 320-30.

FERREIRA, C., BUCCHINI, D., MARTIN, M. E., LEVI, S., AROSIO, P., GRANDCHAMP, B. & BEAUMONT, C. (2000) Early embryonic lethality of H ferritin gene deletion in mice. *J Biol Chem,* 275, 3021-4.

FINCH, R. A., LIU, M., GRILL, S. P., ROSE, W. C., LOOMIS, R., VASQUEZ, K. M., CHENG, Y. & SARTORELLI, A. C. (2000) Triapine (3-aminopyridine-2-carboxaldehyde- thiosemicarbazone): A potent inhibitor of ribonucleotide reductase activity with broad spectrum antitumor activity. *Biochem Pharmacol,* 59, 983-91.

FLORENCE, A. & ATTWOOD, D. (1988) *Physicochemical principles of pharmacy,* London, Macmillan.

FORD, G. C., HARRISON, P. M., RICE, D. W., SMITH, J. M., TREFFRY, A., WHITE, J. L. & YARIV, J. (1984) Ferritin: design and formation of an iron-storage molecule. *Philos Trans R Soc Lond B Biol Sci,* 304, 551-65.

FOURY, F. & CAZZALINI, O. (1997) Deletion of the yeast homologue of the human gene associated with Friedreich's ataxia elicits iron accumulation in mitochondria. *FEBS Lett,* 411, 373-7.

FRAZER, D. M., WILKINS, S. J., VULPE, C. D. & ANDERSON, G. J. (2005) The role of duodenal cytochrome b in intestinal iron absorption remains unclear. *Blood,* 106, 4413; author reply 4414.

FRIEDREICH, N. (1863a) Uber degenerative Atrophie der spinalen Hinterstrange. *Virchow's Arch Pathol Anat,* 27, 1-26.

FRIEDREICH, N. (1863b) Uber degenerative Atrophie der spinalen Hinterstrange. *Virchow's Arch Pathol Anat,* 26, 433-59.

FRIEDREICH, N. (1863c) Uber degenerative Atrophie der spinalen Hinterstrange. *Virchow's Arch Pathol Anat,* 26, 391-419.

FRIEDREICH, N. (1876) Uber ataxie mit besonderer berucksichtigung. *Virchow's Arch Pathol Anat,* 68, 142-245.

FRIEDREICH, N. (1877) Uber ataxie mit besonderer berucksichtigung der hereditaren formen. *Virchow's Arch Pathol Anat,* 70, 140-52.

FUNAKOSHI, N., ONIZUKA, M., YANAGI, K., OHSHIMA, N., TOMOYASU, M., SATO, Y., YAMAMOTO, T., ISHIKAWA, S. & MITSUI, T. (2000) A new model of lung metastasis for intravital studies. *Microvasc Res,* 59, 361-7.

GAETA, A. & HIDER, R. C. (2005) The crucial role of metal ions in neurodegeneration: the basis for a promising therapeutic strategy. *Br J Pharmacol,* 146, 1041-59.

GAKH, O., PARK, S., LIU, G., MACOMBER, L., IMLAY, J. A., FERREIRA, G. C. & ISAYA, G. (2006) Mitochondrial iron detoxification is a primary function of frataxin that limits oxidative damage and preserves cell longevity. *Hum Mol Genet,* 15, 467-79.

GALY, B., FERRING-APPEL, D., KADEN, S., GRONE, H. J. & HENTZE, M. W. (2008) Iron regulatory proteins are essential for intestinal function and control key iron absorption molecules in the duodenum. *Cell Metab,* 7, 79-85.

GALY, B., FERRING, D., MINANA, B., BELL, O., JANSER, H. G., MUCKENTHALER, M., SCHUMANN, K. & HENTZE, M. W. (2005) Altered body iron distribution and microcytosis in mice deficient in iron regulatory protein 2 (IRP2). *Blood,* 106, 2580-9.

GANGOPADHYAY, S., JALALI, F., REDA, D., PEACOCK, J., BRISTOW, R. G. & BENCHIMOL, S. (2002) Expression of different mutant p53 transgenes in neuroblastoma cells leads to different cellular responses to genotoxic agents. *Exp Cell Res,* 275, 122-31.

GANZ, T. & NEMETH, E. (2006) Iron imports. IV. Hepcidin and regulation of body iron metabolism. *Am J Physiol Gastrointest Liver Physiol,* 290, G199-203.

GANZ, T., OLBINA, G., GIRELLI, D., NEMETH, E. & WESTERMAN, M. (2008) Immunoassay for human serum hepcidin. *Blood,* 112, 4292-7.

GAO, J., CHEN, J., DE DOMENICO, I., KOELLER, D. M., HARDING, C. O., FLEMING, R. E., KOEBERL, D. D. & ENNS, C. A. (2010) Hepatocyte-targeted HFE and TFR2 control hepcidin expression in mice. *Blood,* 115, 3374-81.

GAO, J. & RICHARDSON, D. R. (2001) The potential of iron chelators of the pyridoxal isonicotinoyl hydrazone class as effective antiproliferative agents, IV: The mechanisms involved in inhibiting cell-cycle progression. *Blood,* 98, 842-50.

GERBER, J. & LILL, R. (2002) Biogenesis of iron-sulfur proteins in eukaryotes: components, mechanism and pathology. *Mitochondrion, 2,* 71-86.

GIROLAMI, F., HO, C. Y., SEMSARIAN, C., BALDI, M., WILL, M. L., BALDINI, K., TORRICELLI, F., YEATES, L., CECCHI, F., ACKERMAN, M. J. & OLIVOTTO, I. (2010) Clinical features and outcome of hypertrophic cardiomyopathy associated with triple sarcomere protein gene mutations. *J Am Coll Cardiol,* 55, 1444-53.

GLICKSTEIN, H., EL, R. B., LINK, G., BREUER, W., KONIJN, A. M., HERSHKO, C., NICK, H. & CABANTCHIK, Z. I. (2006) Action of chelators in iron-loaded cardiac cells: Accessibility to intracellular labile iron and functional consequences. *Blood,* 108, 3195-203.

GOH, A. M., COFFILL, C. R. & LANE, D. P. (2011) The role of mutant p53 in human cancer. *J Pathol,* 223, 116-26.

GORELL, J. M., ORDIDGE, R. J., BROWN, G. G., DENIAU, J. C., BUDERER, N. M. & HELPERN, J. A. (1995) Increased iron-related MRI contrast in the substantia nigra in Parkinson's disease. *Neurology,* 45, 1138-43.

GOSRIWATANA, I., LOREAL, O., LU, S., BRISSOT, P., PORTER, J. & HIDER, R. C. (1999) Quantification of non-transferrin-bound iron in the presence of unsaturated transferrin. *Anal Biochem,* 273, 212-20.

GOSWAMI, T. & ANDREWS, N. C. (2006) Hereditary hemochromatosis protein, HFE, interaction with transferrin receptor 2 suggests a molecular mechanism for mammalian iron sensing. *J Biol Chem,* 281, 28494-8.

GRAHAM, R. M., REUTENS, G. M., HERBISON, C. E., DELIMA, R. D., CHUA, A. C., OLYNYK, J. K. & TRINDER, D. (2008) Transferrin receptor 2 mediates uptake of transferrin-bound and non-transferrin-bound iron. *J Hepatol,* 48, 327-34.

GRAHAME-SMITH, D. & ARONSON, J. (2006) *Clinical Pharmacology and Drug Therapy,* New York, Oxford Univeristy Press.

GREBENCHTCHIKOV, N., GEURTS-MOESPOT, A. J., KROOT, J. J., DEN HEIJER, M., TJALSMA, H., SWINKELS, D. W. & SWEEP, F. G. (2009) High-sensitive radioimmunoassay for human serum hepcidin. *Br J Haematol,* 146, 317-25.

GREEN, D. A., ANTHOLINE, W. E., WONG, S. J., RICHARDSON, D. R. & CHITAMBAR, C. R. (2001) Inhibition of malignant cell growth by 311, a novel iron chelator of the pyridoxal isonicotinoyl hydrazone class: effect on the R2 subunit of ribonucleotide reductase. *Clin Cancer Res,* 7, 3574-9.

GREENBERG, G. R. & WINTROBE, M. M. (1946) A labile iron pool. *J Biol Chem,* 165, 397.

GREENOUGH, M., PASE, L., VOSKOBOINIK, I., PETRIS, M. J., O'BRIEN, A. W. & CAMAKARIS, J. (2004) Signals regulating trafficking of Menkes (MNK; ATP7A) copper-translocating P-type ATPase in polarized MDCK cells. *Am J Physiol Cell Physiol,* 287, C1463-71.

GUIMARAES, D. P. & HAINAUT, P. (2002) TP53: a key gene in human cancer. *Biochimie,* 84, 83-93.

GUNSHIN, H., MACKENZIE, B., BERGER, U. V., GUNSHIN, Y., ROMERO, M. F., BORON, W. F., NUSSBERGER, S., GOLLAN, J. L. & HEDIGER, M. A. (1997) Cloning and characterization of a mammalian proton-coupled metal-ion transporter. *Nature,* 388, 482-8.

GUNSHIN, H., STARR, C. N., DIRENZO, C., FLEMING, M. D., JIN, J., GREER, E. L., SELLERS, V. M., GALICA, S. M. & ANDREWS, N. C. (2005) Cybrd1 (duodenal cytochrome b) is not necessary for dietary iron absorption in mice. *Blood,* 106, 2879-83.

GUŞET, G., COSTI, S., LAZAR, E., DEMA, A., CORNIANU, M., VERNIC, C. & PAIUSAN, L. (2010) Expression of vascular endothelial growth factor (VEGF) and assessment of microvascular density with CD34 as prognostic markers for endometrial carcinoma. *Rom J Morphol Embryol,* 51, 677-82.

GUTIERREZ, L., LAZARO, F. J., ABADIA, A. R., ROMERO, M. S., QUINTANA, C., PUERTO MORALES, M., PATINO, C. & ARRANZ, R. (2006) Bioinorganic transformations of liver iron deposits observed by tissue magnetic characterisation in a rat model. *J Inorg Biochem,* 100, 1790-9.

GUTIÉRREZ, L., LAZARO, F. J., ABADIA, A. R., ROMERO, M. S., QUINTANA, C., PUERTO MORALES, M., PATINO, C. & ARRANZ, R. (2006) Bioinorganic transformations of liver iron deposits observed by tissue magnetic characterisation in a rat model. *J Inorg Biochem,* 100, 1790-9.

GUTIÉRREZ, L., QUINTANA, C., PATINO, C., BUENO, J., COPPIN, H., ROTH, M. P. & LAZARO, F. J. (2009) Iron speciation study in Hfe knockout mice tissues: magnetic and ultrastructural characterisation. *Biochim Biophys Acta,* 1792, 541-7.

HACKETT, S., CHUA-ANUSORN, W., POOTRAKUL, P. & ST PIERRE, T. G. (2007) The magnetic susceptibilities of iron deposits in thalassaemic spleen tissue. *Biochim Biophys Acta,* 1772, 330-7.

HAGIST, S., SULTMANN, H., MILLONIG, G., HEBLING, U., KIESLICH, D., KUNER, R., BALAGUER, S., SEITZ, H. K., POUSTKA, A. & MUELLER, S. (2009) In vitro-targeted gene identification in patients with hepatitis C using a genome-wide microarray technology. *Hepatology,* 49, 378-86.

HALLIWELL, B. & GUTTERIDGE, J. M. C. (1999) *Free Radicals in Biology and Medicine,* New York, Oxford University Press.

HALLIWELL, B. & GUTTERIDGE, J. M. C. (2007) *Free Radicals in Biology and Medicine*, Claredon Press; Oxford.

HARDING, A. E. (1981) Friedreich's ataxia: a clinical and genetic study of 90 families with an analysis of early diagnostic criteria and intrafamilial clustering of clinical features. *Brain,* 104, 589-620.

HARRIS, D. C. & AISEN, P. (1973) Facilitation of Fe(II) autoxidation by Fe(3) complexing agents. *Biochim Biophys Acta,* 329, 156-8.

HARRISON, P. M. & AROSIO, P. (1996) The ferritins: molecular properties, iron storage function and cellular regulation. *Biochim Biophys Acta,* 1275, 161-203.

HARRISON, P. M., HOY, T. G., MACARA, I. G. & HOARE, R. J. (1974) Ferritin iron uptake and release. Structure-function relationships. *Biochem J,* 143, 445-51.

HASINOFF, B. B., SCHNABL, K. L., MARUSAK, R. A., PATEL, D. & HUEBNER, E. (2003) Dexrazoxane (ICRF-187) protects cardiac myocytes against doxorubicin by preventing damage to mitochondria. *Cardiovasc Toxicol,* 3, 89-99.

HATAKAWA, H., FUNAKOSHI, N., ONIZUKA, M., YANAGI, K., OHSHIMA, N., SATOH, Y., YAMAMOTO, T. & ISHIKAWA, S. (2002) Blood flow does not correlate with the size of metastasis in our new intravital observation model of Lewis lung cancer. *Microvasc Res,* 64, 32-7.

HE, Y., ALAM, S. L., PROTEASA, S. V., ZHANG, Y., LESUISSE, E., DANCIS, A. & STEMMLER, T. L. (2004) Yeast frataxin solution structure, iron binding, and ferrochelatase interaction. *Biochemistry,* 43, 16254-62.

HENTZE, M. W. & KUHN, L. C. (1996) Molecular control of vertebrate iron metabolism: mRNA-based regulatory circuits operated by iron, nitric oxide, and oxidative stress. *Proc Natl Acad Sci U S A,* 93, 8175-82.

HENTZE, M. W., MUCKENTHALER, M. U., GALY, B. & CAMASCHELLA, C. (2010) Two to tango: regulation of Mammalian iron metabolism. *Cell,* 142, 24-38.

HERNANDEZ, O. M., JONES, M., GUZMAN, G. & SZCZESNA-CORDARY, D. (2007) Myosin essential light chain in health and disease. *Am J Physiol Heart Circ Physiol,* 292, H1643-54.

HERSHKO, C., GRAHAM, G., BATES, G. W. & RACHMILEWITZ, E. A. (1978) Non-specific serum iron in thalassaemia: an abnormal serum iron fraction of potential toxicity. *Br J Haematol,* 40, 255-63.

HOLLANDER, D., RICKETTS, D. & BOYD, C. A. R. (1988) Importance of probe molecular geometry in determining intestinal permeability. *Can. J. Gastroenterol,* 2, 35A-38A.

HONDA, K., CASADESUS, G., PETERSEN, R. B., PERRY, G. & SMITH, M. A. (2004) Oxidative stress and redox-active iron in Alzheimer's disease. *Ann N Y Acad Sci,* 1012, 179-82.

HONDA, K., SMITH, M. A., ZHU, X., BAUS, D., MERRICK, W. C., TARTAKOFF, A. M., HATTIER, T., HARRIS, P. L., SIEDLAK, S. L., FUJIOKA, H., LIU, Q., MOREIRA, P. I., MILLER, F. P., NUNOMURA, A., SHIMOHAMA, S. & PERRY, G. (2005) Ribosomal RNA in Alzheimer disease is oxidized by bound redox-active iron. *J Biol Chem,* 280, 20978-86.

HOY, T., HUMPHRYS, J., JACOBS, A., WILLIAMS, A. & PONKA, P. (1979) Effective iron chelation following oral administration of an isoniazid-pyridoxal hydrazone. *Br J Haematol,* 43, 443-9.

HUANG, F. W., PINKUS, J. L., PINKUS, G. S., FLEMING, M. D. & ANDREWS, N. C. (2005) A mouse model of juvenile hemochromatosis. *J Clin Invest,* 115, 2187-91.

HUANG, M. L., BECKER, E. M., WHITNALL, M., RAHMANTO, Y. S., PONKA, P. & RICHARDSON, D. R. (2009) Elucidation of the mechanism of mitochondrial iron loading in Friedreich's ataxia by analysis of a mouse mutant. *Proc Natl Acad Sci U S A,* 106, 16381-6.

IANCU, T. C. (1992) Ferritin and hemosiderin in pathological tissues. *Electron Microsc Rev,* 5, 209-29.

IOFFE, M. L., WHITE, E., NELSON, D. A., DVORZHINSKI, D. & DIPAOLA, R. S. (2004) Epothilone induced cytotoxicity is dependent on p53 status in prostate cells. *Prostate,* 61, 243-7.

JACOBS, A. (1977) Low molecular weight intracellular iron transport compounds. *Blood,* 50, 433-9.

JANSSON, P. J., HAWKINS, C. L., LOVEJOY, D. B. & RICHARDSON, D. R. (2010) The iron complex of Dp44mT is redox-active and induces hydroxyl radical formation: an EPR study. *J Inorg Biochem,* 104, 1224-8.

JEONG, S. Y. & DAVID, S. (2003) Glycosylphosphatidylinositol-anchored ceruloplasmin is required for iron efflux from cells in the central nervous system. *J Biol Chem,* 278, 27144-8.

JEONG, S. Y. & DAVID, S. (2006) Age-related changes in iron homeostasis and cell death in the cerebellum of ceruloplasmin-deficient mice. *J Neurosci,* 26, 9810-9.

JIANG, Z. G., LU, X. C., NELSON, V., YANG, X., PAN, W., CHEN, R. W., LEBOWITZ, M. S., ALMASSIAN, B., TORTELLA, F. C., BRADY, R. O. & GHANBARI, H. A. (2006) A multifunctional cytoprotective agent that reduces neurodegeneration after ischemia. *Proc Natl Acad Sci U S A,* 103, 1581-6.

JOHNSON, D. K., PIPPARD, M. J., MURPHY, T. B. & ROSE, N. J. (1982) An in vivo evaluation of iron-chelating drugs derived from pyridoxal and its analogs. *J Pharmacol Exp Ther,* 221, 399-403.

JONKER, J. W., BUITELAAR, M., WAGENAAR, E., VAN DER VALK, M. A., SCHEFFER, G. L., SCHEPER, R. J., PLOSCH, T., KUIPERS, F., ELFERINK, R. P., ROSING, H., BEIJNEN, J. H. & SCHINKEL, A. H.

(2002) The breast cancer resistance protein protects against a major chlorophyll-derived dietary phototoxin and protoporphyria. *Proc Natl Acad Sci U S A,* 99, 15649-54.

KAKHLON, O., BREUER, W., MUNNICH, A. & CABANTCHIK, Z. I. (2010) Iron redistribution as a therapeutic strategy for treating diseases of localized iron accumulation. *Can J Physiol Pharmacol,* 88, 187-96.

KALINOWSKI, D. S. & RICHARDSON, D. R. (2005) The evolution of iron chelators for the treatment of iron overload disease and cancer. *Pharmacol Rev,* 57, 547-83.

KALINOWSKI, D. S. & RICHARDSON, D. R. (2007) Future of toxicology--iron chelators and differing modes of action and toxicity: the changing face of iron chelation therapy. *Chem Res Toxicol,* 20, 715-20.

KALINOWSKI, D. S., YU, Y., SHARPE, P. C., ISLAM, M., LIAO, Y. T., LOVEJOY, D. B., KUMAR, N., BERNHARDT, P. V. & RICHARDSON, D. R. (2007) Design, synthesis, and characterization of novel iron chelators: structure-activity relationships of the 2-benzoylpyridine thiosemicarbazone series and their 3-nitrobenzoyl analogues as potent antitumor agents. *J Med Chem,* 50, 3716-29.

KATO, J., FUJIKAWA, K., KANDA, M., FUKUDA, N., SASAKI, K., TAKAYAMA, T., KOBUNE, M., TAKADA, K., TAKIMOTO, R., HAMADA, H., IKEDA, T. & NIITSU, Y. (2001) A mutation, in the iron-responsive element of H ferritin mRNA, causing autosomal dominant iron overload. *Am J Hum Genet,* 69, 191-7.

KAWABATA, H., GERMAIN, R. S., IKEZOE, T., TONG, X., GREEN, E. M., GOMBART, A. F. & KOEFFLER, H. P. (2001) Regulation of expression of murine transferrin receptor 2. *Blood,* 98, 1949-54.

KAWABATA, H., YANG, R., HIRAMA, T., VUONG, P. T., KAWANO, S., GOMBART, A. F. & KOEFFLER, H. P. (1999) Molecular cloning of transferrin receptor 2. A new member of the transferrin receptor-like family. *J Biol Chem,* 274, 20826-32.

KIDD, P. M. (2005) Neurodegeneration from mitochondrial insufficiency: nutrients, stem cells, growth factors, and prospects for brain rebuilding using integrative management. *Altern Med Rev,* 10, 268-93.

KIM, B. E., NEVITT, T. & THIELE, D. J. (2008) Mechanisms for copper acquisition, distribution and regulation. *Nat Chem Biol,* 4, 176-85.

KIM, B. E., TURSKI, M. L., NOSE, Y., CASAD, M., ROCKMAN, H. A. & THIELE, D. J. (2010) Cardiac copper deficiency activates a systemic signaling mechanism that communicates with the copper acquisition and storage organs. *Cell Metab,* 11, 353-63.

KISPAL, G., CSERE, P., PROHL, C. & LILL, R. (1999) The mitochondrial proteins Atm1p and Nfs1p are essential for biogenesis of cytosolic Fe/S proteins. *EMBO J,* 18, 3981-9.

KNUTSON, M. D., OUKKA, M., KOSS, L. M., AYDEMIR, F. & WESSLING-RESNICK, M. (2005) Iron release from macrophages after erythrophagocytosis is up-regulated by ferroportin 1 overexpression and down-regulated by hepcidin. *Proc Natl Acad Sci U S A,* 102, 1324-8.

KNUTSON, M. D., VAFA, M. R., HAILE, D. J. & WESSLING-RESNICK, M. (2003) Iron loading and erythrophagocytosis increase ferroportin 1 (FPN1) expression in J774 macrophages. *Blood,* 102, 4191-7.

KOKKINAKIS, D. M., AHMED, M. M., CHENDIL, D., MOSCHEL, R. C. & PEGG, A. E. (2003) Sensitization of pancreatic tumor xenografts to carmustine and temozolomide by inactivation of their O6-Methylguanine-DNA methyltransferase with O6-benzylguanine or O6-benzyl-2'-deoxyguanosine. *Clin Cancer Res,* 9, 3801-7.

KOLB, A. M., SMIT, N. P., LENTZ-LJUBOJE, R., OSANTO, S. & VAN PELT, J. (2009) Non-transferrin bound iron measurement is influenced by chelator concentration. *Anal Biochem,* 385, 13-9.

KOLIARAKI, V., MARINOU, M., VASSILAKOPOULOS, T. P., VAVOURAKIS, E., TSOCHATZIS, E., PANGALIS, G. A., PAPATHEODORIDIS, G., STAMOULAKATOU, A., SWINKELS, D. W., PAPANIKOLAOU, G. & MAMALAKI, A. (2009) A novel immunological assay for hepcidin quantification in human serum. *PLoS One,* 4, e4581.

KONIJN, A. M., GLICKSTEIN, H., VAISMAN, B., MEYRON-HOLTZ, E. G., SLOTKI, I. N. & CABANTCHIK, Z. I. (1999) The cellular labile iron pool and intracellular ferritin in K562 cells. *Blood,* 94, 2128-34.

KOUTNIKOVA, H., CAMPUZANO, V., FOURY, F., DOLLE, P., CAZZALINI, O. & KOENIG, M. (1997) Studies of human, mouse and yeast homologues indicate a mitochondrial function for frataxin. *Nat Genet,* 16, 345-51.

KOVACEVIC, Z., FU, D. & RICHARDSON, D. R. (2008) The iron-regulated metastasis suppressor, Ndrg-1: identification of novel molecular targets. *Biochim Biophys Acta,* 1783, 1981-92.

KRAUSE, A., NEITZ, S., MAGERT, H. J., SCHULZ, A., FORSSMANN, W. G., SCHULZ-KNAPPE, P. & ADERMANN, K. (2000) LEAP-1, a novel highly disulfide-bonded human peptide, exhibits antimicrobial activity. *FEBS Lett,* 480, 147-50.

KROOT, J. J., KEMNA, E. H., BANSAL, S. S., BUSBRIDGE, M., CAMPOSTRINI, N., GIRELLI, D., HIDER, R. C., KOLIARAKI, V., MAMALAKI, A., OLBINA, G., TOMOSUGI, N., TSELEPIS, C., WARD, D. G., GANZ, T., HENDRIKS, J. C. & SWINKELS, D. W. (2009) Results of the first international round robin for the quantification of urinary and plasma hepcidin assays: need for standardization. *Haematologica,* 94, 1748-52.

KUCHAR, J. & HAUSINGER, R. P. (2004) Biosynthesis of metal sites. *Chem Rev,* 104, 509-25.

KUHN, L. C. & HENTZE, M. W. (1992) Coordination of cellular iron metabolism by post-transcriptional gene regulation. *J Inorg Biochem,* 47, 183-95.

KUNINGER, D., KUNS-HASHIMOTO, R., KUZMICKAS, R. & ROTWEIN, P. (2006) Complex biosynthesis of the muscle-enriched iron regulator RGMc. *J Cell Sci,* 119, 3273-83.

KURDISTANI, S. K., ARIZTI, P., REIMER, C. L., SUGRUE, M. M., AARONSON, S. A. & LEE, S. W. (1998) Inhibition of tumor cell growth by RTP/rit42 and its responsiveness to p53 and DNA damage. *Cancer Res,* 58, 4439-44.

KWOK, J. C. & RICHARDSON, D. R. (2002) Unexpected anthracycline-mediated alterations in iron-regulatory protein-RNA-binding activity: the iron and copper complexes of anthracyclines decrease RNA-binding activity. *Mol Pharmacol,* 62, 888-900.

KWOK, J. C. & RICHARDSON, D. R. (2004) Examination of the mechanism(s) involved in doxorubicin-mediated iron accumulation in ferritin: studies using metabolic inhibitors, protein synthesis inhibitors, and lysosomotropic agents. *Mol Pharmacol,* 65, 181-95.

LADAME, P. (1890) Friedreich's disease. *Brain,* 13, 467-537.

LAMARCHE, J., SHAPCOTT, D., COTE, M. & LEMIEUX, B. (1993) Cardiac iron deposits in Friedreich's ataxia. *Handbook of cerebellar diseases.* New York, Marcel Dekker.

LAN, J. & JIANG, D. H. (1997) Desferrioxamine and vitamin E protect against iron and MPTP-induced neurodegeneration in mice. *J Neural Transm,* 104, 469-81.

LAND, T. & ROUAULT, T. A. (1998) Targeting of a human iron-sulfur cluster assembly enzyme, nifs, to different subcellular compartments is regulated through alternative AUG utilization. *Mol Cell,* 2, 807-15.

LANGLOIS D'ESTAINTOT, B., SANTAMBROGIO, P., GRANIER, T., GALLOIS, B., CHEVALIER, J. M., PRECIGOUX, G., LEVI, S. & AROSIO, P. (2004) Crystal structure and biochemical properties of the human mitochondrial ferritin and its mutant Ser144Ala. *J Mol Biol,* 340, 277-93.

LASKEY, J. D., PONKA, P. & SCHULMAN, H. M. (1986) Control of heme synthesis during Friend cell differentiation: role of iron and transferrin. *J Cell Physiol,* 129, 185-92.

LAZARO, F. J., ABADIA, A. R., ROMERO, M. S., GUTIERREZ, L., LAZARO, J. & MORALES, M. P. (2005) Magnetic characterisation of rat muscle tissues after subcutaneous iron dextran injection. *Biochim Biophys Acta,* 1740, 434-45.

LÁZARO, F. J., GUTIÉRREZ, L., ABADÍA, A. R., ROMERO, M. S. & LÓPEZ, A. (2007) Biological tissue magnetism in the frame of iron overload diseases. *Journal of Magnetism and Magnetic Materials,* 316, 126-131.

LE, N. T. & RICHARDSON, D. R. (2002) The role of iron in cell cycle progression and the proliferation of neoplastic cells. *Biochim Biophys Acta,* 1603, 31-46.

LE, N. T. & RICHARDSON, D. R. (2004) Iron chelators with high antiproliferative activity up-regulate the expression of a growth inhibitory and metastasis suppressor gene: a link between iron metabolism and proliferation. *Blood,* 104, 2967-75.

LEE, P. L. & BEUTLER, E. (2009) Regulation of hepcidin and iron-overload disease. *Annu Rev Pathol,* 4, 489-515.

LEIDGENS, S., DE SMET, S. & FOURY, F. (2010) Frataxin interacts with Isu1 through a conserved tryptophan in its beta-sheet. *Hum Mol Genet,* 19, 276-86.

LESUISSE, E., SANTOS, R., MATZANKE, B. F., KNIGHT, S. A., CAMADRO, J. M. & DANCIS, A. (2003) Iron use for haeme synthesis is under control of the yeast frataxin homologue (Yfh1). *Hum Mol Genet,* 12, 879-89.

LEVENSON, C. W. (2003) Iron and Parkinson's disease: chelators to the rescue? *Nutr Rev,* 61, 311-3.

LEVI, S., CORSI, B., BOSISIO, M., INVERNIZZI, R., VOLZ, A., SANFORD, D., AROSIO, P. & DRYSDALE, J. (2001) A human mitochondrial ferritin encoded by an intronless gene. *J Biol Chem*, 276, 24437-40.

LEVI, S., LUZZAGO, A., CESARENI, G., COZZI, A., FRANCESCHINELLI, F., ALBERTINI, A. & AROSIO, P. (1988) Mechanism of ferritin iron uptake: activity of the H-chain and deletion mapping of the ferro-oxidase site. A study of iron uptake and ferro-oxidase activity of human liver, recombinant H-chain ferritins, and of two H-chain deletion mutants. *J Biol Chem*, 263, 18086-92.

LEVI, S. & ROVIDA, E. (2009) The role of iron in mitochondrial function. *Biochim Biophys Acta*, 1790, 629-36.

LI, K., BESSE, E. K., HA, D., KOVTUNOVYCH, G. & ROUAULT, T. A. (2008) Iron-dependent regulation of frataxin expression: implications for treatment of Friedreich ataxia. *Hum Mol Genet*, 17, 2265-73.

LI, Z., ZHANG, H., DONG, X., BURCZYNSKI, F. J., CHOY, P., YANG, F., LIU, H., LI, P. & GONG, Y. (2010) Proteomic profile of primary isolated rat mesangial cells in high-glucose culture condition and decreased expression of PSMA6 in renal cortex of diabetic rats. *Biochem Cell Biol*, 88, 635-48.

LI, Z. Q., OHNO, K. & KAWAZOE, Y. (1996) Structure and Magnetism of Iron-Sulfur Clusters. *Sci. Rep. RITU*, A41, 211-214.

LIANG, S. X. & RICHARDSON, D. R. (2003) The effect of potent iron chelators on the regulation of p53: examination of the expression, localization and DNA-binding activity of p53 and the transactivation of WAF1. *Carcinogenesis*, 24, 1601-14.

LILL, R. & MUHLENHOFF, U. (2008) Maturation of iron-sulfur proteins in eukaryotes: mechanisms, connected processes, and diseases. *Annu Rev Biochem,* 77, 669-700.

LIM, C. K., KALINOWSKI, D. S. & RICHARDSON, D. R. (2008) Protection against hydrogen peroxide-mediated cytotoxicity in Friedreich's ataxia fibroblasts using novel iron chelators of the 2-pyridylcarboxaldehyde isonicotinoyl hydrazone class. *Mol Pharmacol,* 74, 225-35.

LIM, J. E., JIN, O., BENNETT, C., MORGAN, K., WANG, F., TRENOR, C. C., 3RD, FLEMING, M. D. & ANDREWS, N. C. (2005) A mutation in Sec15l1 causes anemia in hemoglobin deficit (hbd) mice. *Nat Genet,* 37, 1270-3.

LIN, L., GOLDBERG, Y. P. & GANZ, T. (2005) Competitive regulation of hepcidin mRNA by soluble and cell-associated hemojuvelin. *Blood,* 106, 2884-9.

LIN, L., NEMETH, E., GOODNOUGH, J. B., THAPA, D. R., GABAYAN, V. & GANZ, T. (2008) Soluble hemojuvelin is released by proprotein convertase-mediated cleavage at a conserved polybasic RNRR site. *Blood Cells Mol Dis,* 40, 122-31.

LINDEN, T., KATSCHINSKI, D. M., ECKHARDT, K., SCHEID, A., PAGEL, H. & WENGER, R. H. (2003) The antimycotic ciclopirox olamine induces HIF-1alpha stability, VEGF expression, and angiogenesis. *FASEB J,* 17, 761-3.

LINDEN, T. & WENGER, R. H. (2003) Iron chelation, angiogenesis and tumor therapy. *Int J Cancer,* 106, 458-9.

LINK, G., PONKA, P., KONIJN, A. M., BREUER, W., CABANTCHIK, Z. I. & HERSHKO, C. (2003) Effects of combined chelation treatment with pyridoxal isonicotinoyl hydrazone analogs and deferoxamine in hypertransfused rats and in iron-loaded rat heart cells. *Blood,* 101, 4172-9.

LIU, Z. D. & HIDER, R. C. (2002) Design of clinically useful iron(III)-selective chelators. *Med Res Rev,* 22, 26-64.

LOCK, R. B., LIEM, N., FARNSWORTH, M. L., MILROSS, C. G., XUE, C., TAJBAKHSH, M., HABER, M., NORRIS, M. D., MARSHALL, G. M. & RICE, A. M. (2002) The nonobese diabetic/severe combined immunodeficient (NOD/SCID) mouse model of childhood acute lymphoblastic leukemia reveals intrinsic differences in biologic characteristics at diagnosis and relapse. *Blood,* 99, 4100-8.

LODI, R., RAJAGOPALAN, B., BRADLEY, J. L., TAYLOR, D. J., CRILLEY, J. G., HART, P. E., BLAMIRE, A. M., MANNERS, D., STYLES, P., SCHAPIRA, A. H. & COOPER, J. M. (2002) Mitochondrial dysfunction in Friedreich's ataxia: from pathogenesis to treatment perspectives. *Free Radic Res,* 36, 461-6.

LOREAL, O., GOSRIWATANA, I., GUYADER, D., PORTER, J., BRISSOT, P. & HIDER, R. C. (2000) Determination of non-transferrin-bound iron in genetic hemochromatosis using a new HPLC-based method. *J Hepatol,* 32, 727-33.

LOWE, S. W. (1995) Cancer therapy and p53. *Curr Opin Oncol,* 7, 547-53.

LU, X., ERRINGTON, J., CURTIN, N. J., LUNEC, J. & NEWELL, D. R. (2001) The impact of p53 status on cellular sensitivity to antifolate drugs. *Clin Cancer Res,* 7, 2114-23.

LYMBOUSSAKI, A., PIGNATTI, E., MONTOSI, G., GARUTI, C., HAILE, D. J. & PIETRANGELO, A. (2003) The role of the iron responsive element in the control of ferroportin1/IREG1/MTP1 gene expression. *J Hepatol,* 39, 710-5.

MADSEN, E. & GITLIN, J. D. (2007) Copper and iron disorders of the brain. *Annu Rev Neurosci,* 30, 317-37.

MAKEYEV, A. V. & LIEBHABER, S. A. (2002) The poly(C)-binding proteins: a multiplicity of functions and a search for mechanisms. *RNA,* 8, 265-78.

MAXTON, D. G., BJARNASON, I., REYNOLDS, A. P., CATT, S. D., PETERS, T. J. & MENZIES, I. S. (1986) Lactulose, 51Cr-labelled ethylenediaminetetra-acetate, L-rhamnose and polyethyleneglycol 400 [corrected] as probe markers for assessment in vivo of human intestinal permeability. *Clin Sci (Lond),* 71, 71-80.

MCCANCE, R. & WIDDOWSON, E. (1938) The absorption and excretion of Fe following oral and intravenous administration. *J Phys,* 94, 148.

MCGUIRE, J. J. (2003) Anticancer antifolates: current status and future directions. *Curr Pharm Des,* 9, 2593-613.

MCKIE, A. T. (2008) The role of Dcytb in iron metabolism: an update. *Biochem Soc Trans,* 36, 1239-41.

MCKIE, A. T., BARROW, D., LATUNDE-DADA, G. O., ROLFS, A., SAGER, G., MUDALY, E., MUDALY, M., RICHARDSON, C., BARLOW, D., BOMFORD, A., PETERS, T. J., RAJA, K. B., SHIRALI, S., HEDIGER, M. A., FARZANEH, F. & SIMPSON, R. J. (2001) An iron-regulated ferric reductase associated with the absorption of dietary iron. *Science,* 291, 1755-9.

MERLE, U., FEIN, E., GEHRKE, S. G., STREMMEL, W. & KULAKSIZ, H. (2007) The iron regulatory peptide hepcidin is expressed in the heart and regulated by hypoxia and inflammation. *Endocrinology,* 148, 2663-8.

MEYRON-HOLTZ, E. G., GHOSH, M. C., IWAI, K., LAVAUTE, T., BRAZZOLOTTO, X., BERGER, U. V., LAND, W., OLLIVIERRE-WILSON, H., GRINBERG, A., LOVE, P. & ROUAULT, T. A. (2004a) Genetic ablations of iron regulatory proteins 1 and 2 reveal why iron regulatory protein 2 dominates iron homeostasis. *EMBO J,* 23, 386-95.

MEYRON-HOLTZ, E. G., GHOSH, M. C. & ROUAULT, T. A. (2004b) Mammalian tissue oxygen levels modulate iron-regulatory protein activities in vivo. *Science,* 306, 2087-90.

MICHAEL, S., PETROCINE, S. V., QIAN, J., LAMARCHE, J. B., KNUTSON, M. D., GARRICK, M. D. & KOEPPEN, A. H. (2006) Iron and iron-responsive proteins in the cardiomyopathy of Friedreich's ataxia. *Cerebellum,* 5, 257-67.

MIMS, M. P. & PRCHAL, J. T. (2005) Divalent metal transporter 1. *Hematology,* 10, 339-45.

MIRANDA, C. J., SANTOS, M. M., OHSHIMA, K., SMITH, J., LI, L., BUNTING, M., COSSEE, M., KOENIG, M., SEQUEIROS, J., KAPLAN, J. & PANDOLFO, M. (2002) Frataxin knockin mouse. *FEBS Lett,* 512, 291-7.

MLADENKA, P., KALINOWSKI, D. S., HASKOVA, P., BOBROVOVA, Z., HRDINA, R., SIMUNEK, T., NACHTIGAL, P., SEMECKY, V.,

VAVROVA, J., HOLECKOVA, M., PALICKA, V., MAZUROVA, Y., JANSSON, P. J. & RICHARDSON, D. R. (2009) The novel iron chelator, 2-pyridylcarboxaldehyde 2-thiophenecarboxyl hydrazone, reduces catecholamine-mediated myocardial toxicity. *Chem Res Toxicol,* 22, 208-17.

MOOS, T. & MORGAN, E. H. (2004) The metabolism of neuronal iron and its pathogenic role in neurological disease: review. *Ann N Y Acad Sci,* 1012, 14-26.

MORGAN, E. (1981) Transferrin biochemistry, physiology, and clinical significance. *Mol Aspects Med,* 4, 1-123.

MUHLENHOFF, U. & LILL, R. (2000) Biogenesis of iron-sulfur proteins in eukaryotes: a novel task of mitochondria that is inherited from bacteria. *Biochim Biophys Acta,* 1459, 370-82.

MUNOZ, M., VILLAR, I. & GARCIA-ERCE, J. A. (2009) An update on iron physiology. *World J Gastroenterol,* 15, 4617-26.

MURAO, N., ISHIGAI, M., YASUNO, H., SHIMONAKA, Y. & ASO, Y. (2007) Simple and sensitive quantification of bioactive peptides in biological matrices using liquid chromatography/selected reaction monitoring mass spectrometry coupled with trichloroacetic acid clean-up. *Rapid Commun Mass Spectrom,* 21, 4033-8.

MURPHY, C. J. & OUDIT, G. Y. (2010) Iron-overload cardiomyopathy: pathophysiology, diagnosis, and treatment. *J Card Fail,* 16, 888-900.

NAPIER, I., PONKA, P. & RICHARDSON, D. R. (2005) Iron trafficking in the mitochondrion: novel pathways revealed by disease. *Blood,* 105, 1867-74.

NAPOLI, E., MORIN, D., BERNHARDT, R., BUCKPITT, A. & CORTOPASSI, G. (2007) Hemin rescues adrenodoxin, heme a and cytochrome oxidase activity in frataxin-deficient oligodendroglioma cells. *Biochim Biophys Acta,* 1772, 773-80.

NEMETH, E. (2010) Targeting the hepcidin-ferroportin axis in the diagnosis and treatment of anemias. *Adv Hematol,* 2010, 750643.

NEMETH, E., PREZA, G. C., JUNG, C. L., KAPLAN, J., WARING, A. J. & GANZ, T. (2006) The N-terminus of hepcidin is essential for its interaction with ferroportin: structure-function study. *Blood,* 107, 328-33.

NEMETH, E., TUTTLE, M. S., POWELSON, J., VAUGHN, M. B., DONOVAN, A., WARD, D. M., GANZ, T. & KAPLAN, J. (2004) Hepcidin regulates cellular iron efflux by binding to ferroportin and inducing its internalization. *Science,* 306, 2090-3.

NIE, G., CHEN, G., SHEFTEL, A. D., PANTOPOULOS, K. & PONKA, P. (2006) In vivo tumor growth is inhibited by cytosolic iron deprivation caused by the expression of mitochondrial ferritin. *Blood,* 108, 2428-34.

NIE, G., SHEFTEL, A. D., KIM, S. F. & PONKA, P. (2005) Overexpression of mitochondrial ferritin causes cytosolic iron depletion and changes cellular iron homeostasis. *Blood,* 105, 2161-7.

NOULSRI, E., RICHARDSON, D. R., LERDWANA, S., FUCHAROEN, S., YAMAGISHI, T., KALINOWSKI, D. S. & PATTANAPANYASAT, K. (2009) Antitumor activity and mechanism of action of the iron chelator, Dp44mT, against leukemic cells. *Am J Hematol,* 84, 170-6.

NURTJAHJA-TJENDRAPUTRA, E., FU, D., PHANG, J. M. & RICHARDSON, D. R. (2007) Iron chelation regulates cyclin D1 expression via the proteasome: a link to iron deficiency-mediated growth suppression. *Blood,* 109, 4045-54.

O'CONNOR, P. M., JACKMAN, J., BAE, I., MYERS, T. G., FAN, S., MUTOH, M., SCUDIERO, D. A., MONKS, A., SAUSVILLE, E. A., WEINSTEIN, J. N., FRIEND, S., FORNACE, A. J., JR. & KOHN, K. W. (1997) Characterization of the p53 tumor suppressor pathway in cell lines of the National Cancer Institute anticancer drug screen and correlations with the growth-inhibitory potency of 123 anticancer agents. *Cancer Res,* 57, 4285-300.

O'HALLORAN, T. V. & CULOTTA, V. C. (2000) Metallochaperones, an intracellular shuttle service for metal ions. *J Biol Chem,* 275, 25057-60.

O'NEILL, H. A., GAKH, O., PARK, S., CUI, J., MOONEY, S. M., SAMPSON, M., FERREIRA, G. C. & ISAYA, G. (2005) Assembly of human frataxin is a mechanism for detoxifying redox-active iron. *Biochemistry,* 44, 537-45.

OLDENDORF, W. H. (1974) Lipid solubility and drug penetration of the blood brain barrier. *Proc Soc Exp Biol Med,* 147, 813-5.

OLIVIERI, N. F. & BRITTENHAM, G. M. (1997) Iron-chelating therapy and the treatment of thalassemia. *Blood,* 89, 739-61.

PANDOLFO, M. (2003) Friedreich ataxia. *Semin Pediatr Neurol,* 10, 163-72.

PANDOLFO, M. & PASTORE, A. (2009) The pathogenesis of Friedreich ataxia and the structure and function of frataxin. *J Neurol,* 256 Suppl 1, 9-17.

PAPANIKOLAOU, G., SAMUELS, M. E., LUDWIG, E. H., MACDONALD, M. L., FRANCHINI, P. L., DUBE, M. P., ANDRES, L., MACFARLANE, J., SAKELLAROPOULOS, N., POLITOU, M., NEMETH, E., THOMPSON, J., RISLER, J. K., ZABOROWSKA, C., BABAKAIFF, R., RADOMSKI, C. C., PAPE, T. D., DAVIDAS, O., CHRISTAKIS, J., BRISSOT, P., LOCKITCH, G., GANZ, T., HAYDEN, M. R. & GOLDBERG, Y. P. (2004) Mutations in HFE2 cause iron overload in chromosome 1q-linked juvenile hemochromatosis. *Nat Genet,* 36, 77-82.

PARADKAR, P. N., ZUMBRENNEN, K. B., PAW, B. H., WARD, D. M. & KAPLAN, J. (2009) Regulation of mitochondrial iron import through differential turnover of mitoferrin 1 and mitoferrin 2. *Mol Cell Biol,* 29, 1007-16.

PARK, C. H., VALORE, E. V., WARING, A. J. & GANZ, T. (2001) Hepcidin, a urinary antimicrobial peptide synthesized in the liver. *J Biol Chem,* 276, 7806-10.

PARK, J. H., KIM, T. Y., JONG, H. S., CHUN, Y. S., PARK, J. W., LEE, C. T., JUNG, H. C., KIM, N. K. & BANG, Y. J. (2003) Gastric epithelial reactive oxygen species prevent normoxic degradation of hypoxia-inducible factor-1alpha in gastric cancer cells. *Clin Cancer Res,* 9, 433-40.

PARK, S., GAKH, O., MOONEY, S. M. & ISAYA, G. (2002) The ferroxidase activity of yeast frataxin. *J Biol Chem,* 277, 38589-95.

PESLOVA, G., PETRAK, J., KUZELOVA, K., HRDY, I., HALADA, P., KUCHEL, P. W., SOE-LIN, S., PONKA, P., SUTAK, R., BECKER, E., HUANG, M. L., RAHMANTO, Y. S., RICHARDSON, D. R. &

VYORAL, D. (2009) Hepcidin, the hormone of iron metabolism, is bound specifically to alpha-2-macroglobulin in blood. *Blood,* 113, 6225-36.

PETRAK, J. V. & VYORAL, D. (2001) Detection of iron-containing proteins contributing to the cellular labile iron pool by a native electrophoresis metal blotting technique. *J Inorg Biochem,* 86, 669-75.

PEYSSONNAUX, C., ZINKERNAGEL, A. S., SCHUEPBACH, R. A., RANKIN, E., VAULONT, S., HAASE, V. H., NIZET, V. & JOHNSON, R. S. (2007) Regulation of iron homeostasis by the hypoxia-inducible transcription factors (HIFs). *J Clin Invest,* 117, 1926-32.

PIETRANGELO, A. (2010) Hepcidin in human iron disorders: therapeutic implications. *J Hepatol,* 54, 173-81.

PIGA, A., ROGGERO, S., SALUSSOLIA, I., MASSANO, D., SERRA, M. & LONGO, F. (2010) Deferiprone. *Ann N Y Acad Sci,* 1202, 75-8.

PIGEON, C., ILYIN, G., COURSELAUD, B., LEROYER, P., TURLIN, B., BRISSOT, P. & LOREAL, O. (2001) A new mouse liver-specific gene, encoding a protein homologous to human antimicrobial peptide hepcidin, is overexpressed during iron overload. *J Biol Chem,* 276, 7811-9.

POLI, M., LUSCIETI, S., GANDINI, V., MACCARINELLI, F., FINAZZI, D., SILVESTRI, L., ROETTO, A. & AROSIO, P. (2010) Transferrin receptor 2 and HFE regulate furin expression via mitogen-activated protein kinase/extracellular signal-regulated kinase (MAPK/Erk) signaling. Implications for transferrin-dependent hepcidin regulation. *Haematologica,* 95, 1832-40.

POLLA, B. S. (1999) Therapy by taking away: the case of iron. *Biochem Pharmacol,* 57, 1345-9.

PONKA, P. (1997) Tissue-specific regulation of iron metabolism and heme synthesis: distinct control mechanisms in erythroid cells. *Blood,* 89, 1-25.

PONKA, P., BEAUMONT, C. & RICHARDSON, D. R. (1998) Function and regulation of transferrin and ferritin. *Semin Hematol,* 35, 35-54.

PONKA, P., BOROVA, J., NEUWIRT, J. & FUCHS, O. (1979a) Mobilization of iron from reticulocytes. Identification of pyridoxal isonicotinoyl hydrazone as a new iron chelating agent. *FEBS Lett,* 97, 317-21.

PONKA, P., BOROVA, J., NEUWIRT, J., FUCHS, O. & NECAS, E. (1979b) A study of intracellular iron metabolism using pyridoxal isonicotinoyl hydrazone and other synthetic chelating agents. *Biochim Biophys Acta,* 586, 278-97.

PONKA, P., RICHARDSON, D. R., EDWARD, J. T. & CHUBB, F. L. (1994) Iron chelators of the pyridoxal isonicotinoyl hydrazone class. Relationship of the lipophilicity of the apochelator to its ability to mobilise iron from reticulocytes in vitro. *Can J Physiol Pharmacol,* 72, 659-66.

PONKA, P. & SCHULMAN, H. M. (1985) Acquisition of iron from transferrin regulates reticulocyte heme synthesis. *J Biol Chem,* 260, 14717-21.

POPESCU, B. F., PICKERING, I. J., GEORGE, G. N. & NICHOL, H. (2007) The chemical form of mitochondrial iron in Friedreich's ataxia. *J Inorg Biochem,* 101, 957-66.

PUCCIO, H. (2009) Multicellular models of Friedreich ataxia. *J Neurol,* 256 Suppl 1, 18-24.

PUCCIO, H., SIMON, D., COSSEE, M., CRIQUI-FILIPE, P., TIZIANO, F., MELKI, J., HINDELANG, C., MATYAS, R., RUSTIN, P. & KOENIG, M. (2001) Mouse models for Friedreich ataxia exhibit cardiomyopathy, sensory nerve defect and Fe-S enzyme deficiency followed by intramitochondrial iron deposits. *Nat Genet,* 27, 181-6.

PUFAHL, R. A., SINGER, C. P., PEARISO, K. L., LIN, S. J., SCHMIDT, P. J., FAHRNI, C. J., CULOTTA, V. C., PENNER-HAHN, J. E. & O'HALLORAN, T. V. (1997) Metal ion chaperone function of the soluble Cu(I) receptor Atx1. *Science,* 278, 853-6.

QUIGLEY, J. G., YANG, Z., WORTHINGTON, M. T., PHILLIPS, J. D., SABO, K. M., SABATH, D. E., BERG, C. L., SASSA, S., WOOD, B. L. & ABKOWITZ, J. L. (2004) Identification of a human heme exporter that is essential for erythropoiesis. *Cell,* 118, 757-66.

QUINTANA, C. (2007) Contribution of analytical microscopies to human neurodegenerative diseases research (PSP and AD). *Mini Rev Med Chem,* 7, 961-75.

RADISKY, D. C., BABCOCK, M. C. & KAPLAN, J. (1999) The yeast frataxin homologue mediates mitochondrial iron efflux. Evidence for a mitochondrial iron cycle. *J Biol Chem,* 274, 4497-9.

RAE, T. D., SCHMIDT, P. J., PUFAHL, R. A., CULOTTA, V. C. & O'HALLORAN, T. V. (1999) Undetectable intracellular free copper: the requirement of a copper chaperone for superoxide dismutase. *Science,* 284, 805-8.

RAI, M., SORAGNI, E., JENSSEN, K., BURNETT, R., HERMAN, D., COPPOLA, G., GESCHWIND, D. H., GOTTESFELD, J. M. & PANDOLFO, M. (2008) HDAC inhibitors correct frataxin deficiency in a Friedreich ataxia mouse model. *PLoS One,* 3, e1958.

RAO, V. A., KLEIN, S. R., AGAMA, K. K., TOYODA, E., ADACHI, N., POMMIER, Y. & SHACTER, E. B. (2009) The iron chelator Dp44mT causes DNA damage and selective inhibition of topoisomerase IIalpha in breast cancer cells. *Cancer Res,* 69, 948-57.

RICHARDSON, D. R. (2003) Friedreich's ataxia: iron chelators that target the mitochondrion as a therapeutic strategy? *Expert Opin Investig Drugs,* 12, 235-45.

RICHARDSON, D. R. (2005) Molecular mechanisms of iron uptake by cells and the use of iron chelators for the treatment of cancer. *Curr Med Chem,* 12, 2711-29.

RICHARDSON, D. R. & BAKER, E. (1990) The uptake of iron and transferrin by the human malignant melanoma cell. *Biochim Biophys Acta,* 1053, 1-12.

RICHARDSON, D. R. & BAKER, E. (1992) Intermediate steps in cellular iron uptake from transferrin. Detection of a cytoplasmic pool of iron, free of transferrin. *J Biol Chem,* 267, 21384-9.

RICHARDSON, D. R. & BERNHARDT, P. V. (1999) Crystal and molecular structure of 2-hydroxy-1-naphthaldehyde isonicotinoyl hydrazone (NIH) and its iron(III) complex: an iron chelator with anti-tumour activity. *J Biol Inorg Chem,* 4, 266-73.

RICHARDSON, D. R., HEFTER, G. T., MAY, P. M., WEBB, J. & BAKER, E. (1989) Iron chelators of the pyridoxal isonicotinoyl hydrazone class. III. Formation constants with calcium(II), magnesium(II) and zinc(II). *Biol Met,* 2, 161-7.

RICHARDSON, D. R., KALINOWSKI, D. S., LAU, S., JANSSON, P. J. & LOVEJOY, D. B. (2009) Cancer cell iron metabolism and the development of potent iron chelators as anti-tumour agents. *Biochim Biophys Acta,* 1790, 702-17.

RICHARDSON, D. R., LANE, D. J., BECKER, E. M., HUANG, M. L., WHITNALL, M., RAHMANTO, Y. S., SHEFTEL, A. D. & PONKA, P. (2010) Mitochondrial iron trafficking and the integration of iron metabolism between the mitochondrion and cytosol. *Proc Natl Acad Sci U S A,* 107, 10775-82.

RICHARDSON, D. R. & MILNES, K. (1997) The potential of iron chelators of the pyridoxal isonicotinoyl hydrazone class as effective antiproliferative agents II: the mechanism of action of ligands derived from salicylaldehyde benzoyl hydrazone and 2-hydroxy-1-naphthylaldehyde benzoyl hydrazone. *Blood,* 89, 3025-38.

RICHARDSON, D. R., MOURALIAN, C., PONKA, P. & BECKER, E. (2001) Development of potential iron chelators for the treatment of Friedreich's ataxia: ligands that mobilize mitochondrial iron. *Biochim Biophys Acta,* 1536, 133-40.

RICHARDSON, D. R. & PONKA, P. (1997) The molecular mechanisms of the metabolism and transport of iron in normal and neoplastic cells. *Biochim Biophys Acta,* 1331, 1-40.

RICHARDSON, D. R. & PONKA, P. (1998) Pyridoxal isonicotinoyl hydrazone and its analogs: potential orally effective iron-chelating agents for the treatment of iron overload disease. *J Lab Clin Med,* 131, 306-15.

RICHARDSON, D. R., PONKA, P. & VYORAL, D. (1996) Distribution of iron in reticulocytes after inhibition of heme synthesis with succinylacetone: examination of the intermediates involved in iron metabolism. *Blood,* 87, 3477-88.

RICHARDSON, D. R., SHARPE, P. C., LOVEJOY, D. B., SENARATNE, D., KALINOWSKI, D. S., ISLAM, M. & BERNHARDT, P. V. (2006) Dipyridyl thiosemicarbazone chelators with potent and selective antitumor activity form iron complexes with redox activity. *J Med Chem,* 49, 6510-21.

RICHARDSON, D. R., TRAN, E. H. & PONKA, P. (1995) The potential of iron chelators of the pyridoxal isonicotinoyl hydrazone class as effective antiproliferative agents. *Blood,* 86, 4295-306.

RICHARDSON, D. R., VITOLO, L., HEFTER, G. T., MAT, P. M., CLARE, B. W., WEBB, J. & WILAIRAT, P. (1990a) Iron chelators of the pyridoxal isonicotinoyl hydrazone class. Part I. Ionisation characteristics of the ligand and their relevance to biological properties. *Inorg Chim Acta,* 170, 165-170.

RICHARDSON, D. R., WIS VITOLO, L. M., HEFTER, G. T., MAY, P. M., CLARE, B. W., WEBB, J. & WILAIRAT, P. (1990b) Iron chelators of the pyridoxal isonicotinoyl hydrazone class Part I. Ionization characteristics of the ligands and their relevance to biological properties. *Inorg. Chim. Acta,* 170, 165-170.

RISTOW, M., MULDER, H., POMPLUN, D., SCHULZ, T. J., MULLER-SCHMEHL, K., KRAUSE, A., FEX, M., PUCCIO, H., MULLER, J., ISKEN, F., SPRANGER, J., MULLER-WIELAND, D., MAGNUSON, M. A., MOHLIG, M., KOENIG, M. & PFEIFFER, A. F. (2003) Frataxin deficiency in pancreatic islets causes diabetes due to loss of beta cell mass. *J Clin Invest,* 112, 527-34.

ROBB, A. & WESSLING-RESNICK, M. (2004) Regulation of transferrin receptor 2 protein levels by transferrin. *Blood,* 104, 4294-9.

RODRIGUEZ, A., HILVO, M., KYTOMAKI, L., FLEMING, R. E., BRITTON, R. S., BACON, B. R. & PARKKILA, S. (2007) Effects of iron loading on muscle: genome-wide mRNA expression profiling in the mouse. *BMC Genomics,* 8, 379.

ROGERS, J. T., RANDALL, J. D., CAHILL, C. M., EDER, P. S., HUANG, X., GUNSHIN, H., LEITER, L., MCPHEE, J., SARANG, S. S., UTSUKI, T., GREIG, N. H., LAHIRI, D. K., TANZI, R. E., BUSH, A. I., GIORDANO, T. & GULLANS, S. R. (2002) An iron-responsive element type II in the 5'-untranslated region of the Alzheimer's amyloid precursor protein transcript. *J Biol Chem,* 277, 45518-28.

ROSSNER, M. J., HIRRLINGER, J., WICHERT, S. P., BOEHM, C., NEWRZELLA, D., HIEMISCH, H., EISENHARDT, G., STUENKEL, C., VON AHSEN, O. & NAVE, K. A. (2006) Global transcriptome analysis of genetically identified neurons in the adult cortex. *J Neurosci,* 26, 9956-66.

RÖTIG, A., DE LONLAY, P., CHRETIEN, D., FOURY, F., KOENIG, M., SIDI, D., MUNNICH, A. & RUSTIN, P. (1997) Aconitase and mitochondrial iron-sulphur protein deficiency in Friedreich ataxia. *Nat Genet,* 17, 215-7.

ROUAULT, T. & KLAUSNER, R. (1997) Regulation of iron metabolism in eukaryotes. *Curr Top Cell Regul,* 35, 1-19.

ROUAULT, T. A. (2006) The role of iron regulatory proteins in mammalian iron homeostasis and disease. *Nat Chem Biol,* 2, 406-14.

ROUAULT, T. A. (2009) Cell biology. An ancient gauge for iron. *Science,* 326, 676-7.

ROUAULT, T. A., TANG, C. K., KAPTAIN, S., BURGESS, W. H., HAILE, D. J., SAMANIEGO, F., MCBRIDE, O. W., HARFORD, J. B. & KLAUSNER, R. D. (1990) Cloning of the cDNA encoding an RNA regulatory protein--the human iron-responsive element-binding protein. *Proc Natl Acad Sci U S A,* 87, 7958-62.

ROUAULT, T. A. & TONG, W. H. (2008) Iron-sulfur cluster biogenesis and human disease. *Trends Genet,* 24, 398-407.

RUCKER, P., TORTI, F. M. & TORTI, S. V. (1996) Role of H and L subunits in mouse ferritin. *J Biol Chem,* 271, 33352-7.

RÜFENACHT, U. B., GOUYA, L., SCHNEIDER-YIN, X., PUY, H., SCHAFER, B. W., AQUARON, R., NORDMANN, Y., MINDER, E. I. & DEYBACH, J. C. (1998) Systematic analysis of molecular defects in the ferrochelatase gene from patients with erythropoietic protoporphyria. *Am J Hum Genet,* 62, 1341-52.

RUSTIN, P., VON KLEIST-RETZOW, J. C., CHANTREL-GROUSSARD, K., SIDI, D., MUNNICH, A. & ROTIG, A. (1999) Effect of idebenone on cardiomyopathy in Friedreich's ataxia: a preliminary study. *Lancet,* 354, 477-9.

RYVLIN, P., BROUSSOLLE, E., PIOLLET, H., VIALLET, F., KHALFALLAH, Y. & CHAZOT, G. (1995) Magnetic resonance imaging evidence of decreased putamenal iron content in idiopathic Parkinson's disease. *Arch Neurol,* 52, 583-8.

SAAD, S. Y., NAJJAR, T. A. & AL-RIKABI, A. C. (2001) The preventive role of deferoxamine against acute doxorubicin-induced cardiac, renal and hepatic toxicity in rats. *Pharmacol Res,* 43, 211-8.

SAMANIEGO, F., CHIN, J., IWAI, K., ROUAULT, T. A. & KLAUSNER, R. D. (1994) Molecular characterization of a second iron-responsive element binding protein, iron regulatory protein 2. Structure, function, and post-translational regulation. *J Biol Chem,* 269, 30904-10.

SANCHEZ-CASIS, G., COTE, M. & BARBEAU, A. (1976) Pathology of the heart in Friedreich's ataxia: review of the literature and report of one case. *Can J Neurol Sci,* 3, 349-54.

SANTAMBROGIO, P., BIASIOTTO, G., SANVITO, F., OLIVIERI, S., AROSIO, P. & LEVI, S. (2007) Mitochondrial ferritin expression in adult mouse tissues. *J Histochem Cytochem,* 55, 1129-37.

SANTAMBROGIO, P., LEVI, S., COZZI, A., CORSI, B. & AROSIO, P. (1996) Evidence that the specificity of iron incorporation into homopolymers of human ferritin L- and H-chains is conferred by the nucleation and ferroxidase centres. *Biochem J,* 314 (Pt 1), 139-44.

SANTOS, R., LEFEVRE, S., SLIWA, D., SEGUIN, A., CAMADRO, J. M. & LESUISSE, E. (2010) Friedreich ataxia: molecular mechanisms, redox considerations, and therapeutic opportunities. *Antioxid Redox Signal,* 13, 651-90.

SCHNEIDER, E., HORTON, J. K., YANG, C. H., NAKAGAWA, M. & COWAN, K. H. (1994) Multidrug resistance-associated protein gene overexpression and reduced drug sensitivity of topoisomerase II in a human breast carcinoma MCF7 cell line selected for etoposide resistance. *Cancer Res,* 54, 152-8.

SCHOENFELD, R. A., NAPOLI, E., WONG, A., ZHAN, S., REUTENAUER, L., MORIN, D., BUCKPITT, A. R., TARONI, F., LONNERDAL, B., RISTOW, M., PUCCIO, H. & CORTOPASSI, G. A. (2005) Frataxin deficiency alters heme pathway transcripts and decreases mitochondrial heme metabolites in mammalian cells. *Hum Mol Genet,* 14, 3787-99.

SCHULZ, J. B., DEHMER, T., SCHOLS, L., MENDE, H., HARDT, C., VORGERD, M., BURK, K., MATSON, W., DICHGANS, J., BEAL, M. F. & BOGDANOV, M. B. (2000) Oxidative stress in patients with Friedreich ataxia. *Neurology,* 55, 1719-21.

SCHWARZ, P., STRNAD, P., VON FIGURA, G., JANETZKO, A., KRAYENBUHL, P., ADLER, G. & KULAKSIZ, H. (2010) A novel monoclonal antibody immunoassay for the detection of human serum hepcidin. *J Gastroenterol.*

SEKYERE, E. O., DUNN, L. L., RAHMANTO, Y. S. & RICHARDSON, D. R. (2006) Role of melanotransferrin in iron metabolism: studies using targeted gene disruption in vivo. *Blood,* 107, 2599-601.

SEZNEC, H., SIMON, D., BOUTON, C., REUTENAUER, L., HERTZOG, A., GOLIK, P., PROCACCIO, V., PATEL, M., DRAPIER,

J. C., KOENIG, M. & PUCCIO, H. (2005) Friedreich ataxia: the oxidative stress paradox. *Hum Mol Genet,* 14, 463-74.

SEZNEC, H., SIMON, D., MONASSIER, L., CRIQUI-FILIPE, P., GANSMULLER, A., RUSTIN, P., KOENIG, M. & PUCCIO, H. (2004) Idebenone delays the onset of cardiac functional alteration without correction of Fe-S enzymes deficit in a mouse model for Friedreich ataxia. *Hum Mol Genet,* 13, 1017-24.

SHARP, P. & SRAI, S. K. (2007) Molecular mechanisms involved in intestinal iron absorption. *World J Gastroenterol,* 13, 4716-24.

SHAW, G. C., COPE, J. J., LI, L., CORSON, K., HERSEY, C., ACKERMANN, G. E., GWYNN, B., LAMBERT, A. J., WINGERT, R. A., TRAVER, D., TREDE, N. S., BARUT, B. A., ZHOU, Y., MINET, E., DONOVAN, A., BROWNLIE, A., BALZAN, R., WEISS, M. J., PETERS, L. L., KAPLAN, J., ZON, L. I. & PAW, B. H. (2006) Mitoferrin is essential for erythroid iron assimilation. *Nature,* 440, 96-100.

SHAYEGHI, M., LATUNDE-DADA, G. O., OAKHILL, J. S., LAFTAH, A. H., TAKEUCHI, K., HALLIDAY, N., KHAN, Y., WARLEY, A., MCCANN, F. E., HIDER, R. C., FRAZER, D. M., ANDERSON, G. J., VULPE, C. D., SIMPSON, R. J. & MCKIE, A. T. (2005) Identification of an intestinal heme transporter. *Cell,* 122, 789-801.

SHEFTEL, A. D. & LILL, R. (2009) The power plant of the cell is also a smithy: the emerging role of mitochondria in cellular iron homeostasis. *Ann Med,* 41, 82-99.

SHEFTEL, A. D., ZHANG, A. S., BROWN, C., SHIRIHAI, O. S. & PONKA, P. (2007) Direct interorganellar transfer of iron from endosome to mitochondrion. *Blood,* 110, 125-32.

SHEN, D. W., CARDARELLI, C., HWANG, J., CORNWELL, M., RICHERT, N., ISHII, S., PASTAN, I. & GOTTESMAN, M. M. (1986) Multiple drug-resistant human KB carcinoma cells independently selected for high-level resistance to colchicine, adriamycin, or vinblastine show changes in expression of specific proteins. *J Biol Chem,* 261, 7762-70.

SHI, H., BENCZE, K. Z., STEMMLER, T. L. & PHILPOTT, C. C. (2008) A cytosolic iron chaperone that delivers iron to ferritin. *Science,* 320, 1207-10.

SHIRIHAI, O. S., GREGORY, T., YU, C., ORKIN, S. H. & WEISS, M. J. (2000) ABC-me: a novel mitochondrial transporter induced by GATA-1 during erythroid differentiation. *EMBO J,* 19, 2492-502.

SHVARTSMAN, M., KIKKERI, R., SHANZER, A. & CABANTCHIK, Z. I. (2007) Non-transferrin-bound iron reaches mitochondria by a chelator-inaccessible mechanism: biological and clinical implications. *Am J Physiol Cell Physiol,* 293, C1383-94.

SILVESTRI, L., PAGANI, A. & CAMASCHELLA, C. (2008) Furin-mediated release of soluble hemojuvelin: a new link between hypoxia and iron homeostasis. *Blood,* 111, 924-31.

SIMON, D., SEZNEC, H., GANSMULLER, A., CARELLE, N., WEBER, P., METZGER, D., RUSTIN, P., KOENIG, M. & PUCCIO, H. (2004) Friedreich ataxia mouse models with progressive cerebellar and sensory ataxia reveal autophagic neurodegeneration in dorsal root ganglia. *J Neurosci,* 24, 1987-95.

SIPE, J. C., LEE, P. & BEUTLER, E. (2002) Brain iron metabolism and neurodegenerative disorders. *Dev Neurosci,* 24, 188-96.

SMITH, M. A., HARRIS, P. L., SAYRE, L. M. & PERRY, G. (1997) Iron accumulation in Alzheimer disease is a source of redox-generated free radicals. *Proc Natl Acad Sci U S A,* 94, 9866-8.

SMITH, S. R., GHOSH, M. C., OLLIVIERRE-WILSON, H., HANG TONG, W. & ROUAULT, T. A. (2006) Complete loss of iron regulatory proteins 1 and 2 prevents viability of murine zygotes beyond the blastocyst stage of embryonic development. *Blood Cells Mol Dis,* 36, 283-7.

SNYDER, A. M., NEELY, E. B., LEVI, S., AROSIO, P. & CONNOR, J. R. (2010) Regional and cellular distribution of mitochondrial ferritin in the mouse brain. *J Neurosci Res,* 88, 3133-43.

SPROULE, T. J., JAZWINSKA, E. C., BRITTON, R. S., BACON, B. R., FLEMING, R. E., SLY, W. S. & ROOPENIAN, D. C. (2001) Naturally variant autosomal and sex-linked loci determine the severity of iron overload in beta 2-microglobulin-deficient mice. *Proc Natl Acad Sci U S A,* 98, 5170-4.

ST PIERRE, T. G., CHUA-ANUSORN, W., WEBB, J., MACEY, D. & POOTRAKUL, P. (1998) The form of iron oxide deposits in thalassemic tissues varies between different groups of patients: a comparison between Thai beta-thalassemia/hemoglobin E patients and Australian beta-thalassemia patients. *Biochim Biophys Acta,* 1407, 51-60.

STARIAT, J., KOVARIKOVA, P., KLIMES, J., LOVEJOY, D. B., KALINOWSKI, D. S. & RICHARDSON, D. R. (2009) HPLC methods for determination of two novel thiosemicarbazone anti-cancer drugs

(N4mT and Dp44mT) in plasma and their application to in vitro plasma stability of these agents. *J Chromatogr B Analyt Technol Biomed Life Sci,* 877, 316-22.

STEMMLER, T. L., LESUISSE, E., PAIN, D. & DANCIS, A. (2010) Frataxin and mitochondrial FeS cluster biogenesis. *J Biol Chem,* 285, 26737-43.

STURM, B., STUPPHANN, D., KAUN, C., BOESCH, S., SCHRANZHOFER, M., WOJTA, J., GOLDENBERG, H. & SCHEIBER-MOJDEHKAR, B. (2005) Recombinant human erythropoietin: effects on frataxin expression in vitro. *Eur J Clin Invest,* 35, 711-7.

SUTAK, R., XU, X., WHITNALL, M., KASHEM, M. A., VYORAL, D. & RICHARDSON, D. R. (2008) Proteomic analysis of hearts from frataxin knockout mice: marked rearrangement of energy metabolism, a response to cellular stress and altered expression of proteins involved in cell structure, motility and metabolism. *Proteomics,* 8, 1731-41.

SUTHERLAND, R., DELIA, D., SCHNEIDER, C., NEWMAN, R., KEMSHEAD, J. & GREAVES, M. (1981) Ubiquitous cell-surface glycoprotein on tumor cells is proliferation-associated receptor for transferrin. *Proc Natl Acad Sci U S A,* 78, 4515-9.

SWINKELS, D. W., GIRELLI, D., LAARAKKERS, C., KROOT, J., CAMPOSTRINI, N., KEMNA, E. H. & TJALSMA, H. (2008) Advances in quantitative hepcidin measurements by time-of-flight mass spectrometry. *PLoS One,* 3, e2706.

TAETLE, R. & HONEYSETT, J. M. (1987) Effects of monoclonal anti-transferrin receptor antibodies on in vitro growth of human solid tumor cells. *Cancer Res,* 47, 2040-4.

THEIL, E. C. & EISENSTEIN, R. S. (2000) Combinatorial mRNA regulation: iron regulatory proteins and iso-iron-responsive elements (Iso-IREs). *J Biol Chem,* 275, 40659-62.

THELANDER, L. & REICHARD, P. (1979) Reduction of ribonucleotides. *Annu Rev Biochem,* 48, 133-58.

THOMAS, M. & JANKOVIC, J. (2004) Neurodegenerative disease and iron storage in the brain. *Curr Opin Neurol,* 17, 437-42.

THOMPSON, K., MENZIES, S., MUCKENTHALER, M., TORTI, F. M., WOOD, T., TORTI, S. V., HENTZE, M. W., BEARD, J. & CONNOR, J. (2003) Mouse brains deficient in H-ferritin have normal iron concentration but a protein profile of iron deficiency and increased evidence of oxidative stress. *J Neurosci Res,* 71, 46-63.

TILLBROOK, G. S. & HIDER, R. C. (1998) Iron chelators for clinical use. IN A, S. & H, S. (Eds.) *Metal irons in biological systems.* New York, Marcel Dekker.

TOYOZUMI, Y., ARIMA, N., IZUMARU, S., KATO, S., MORIMATSU, M. & NAKASHIMA, T. (2004) Loss of caspase-8 activation pathway is a possible mechanism for CDDP resistance in human laryngeal squamous cell carcinoma, HEp-2 cells. *Int J Oncol,* 25, 721-8.

TRINDER, D., ZAK, O. & AISEN, P. (1996) Transferrin receptor-independent uptake of differic transferrin by human hepatoma cells with antisense inhibition of receptor expression. *Hepatology,* 23, 1512-20.

TROADEC, M. B., WARD, D. M., LO, E., KAPLAN, J. & DE DOMENICO, I. (2010) Induction of FPN1 transcription by MTF-1 reveals a role for ferroportin in transition metal efflux. *Blood,* 116, 4657-64.

TROWBRIDGE, I. S. & LOPEZ, F. (1982) Monoclonal antibody to transferrin receptor blocks transferrin binding and inhibits human tumor cell growth in vitro. *Proc Natl Acad Sci U S A,* 79, 1175-9.

TRUKSA, J., PENG, H., LEE, P. & BEUTLER, E. (2007) Different regulatory elements are required for response of hepcidin to interleukin-6 and bone morphogenetic proteins 4 and 9. *Br J Haematol,* 139, 138-47.

TSE, J. C. & KALLURI, R. (2007) Mechanisms of metastasis: epithelial-to-mesenchymal transition and contribution of tumor microenvironment. *J Cell Biochem,* 101, 816-29.

USUDA, J., INOMATA, M., FUKUMOTO, H., IWAMOTO, Y., SUZUKI, T., KUH, H. J., FUKUOKA, K., KATO, H., SAIJO, N. & NISHIO, K. (2003) Restoration of p53 gene function in 12-O-tetradecanoylphorbor 13-acetate-resistant human leukemia K562/TPA cells. *Int J Oncol,* 22, 81-6.

VALORE, E. V. & GANZ, T. (2008) Posttranslational processing of hepcidin in human hepatocytes is mediated by the prohormone convertase furin. *Blood Cells Mol Dis,* 40, 132-8.

VAN DRIEST, S. L., GAKH, O., OMMEN, S. R., ISAYA, G. & ACKERMAN, M. J. (2005) Molecular and functional characterization of a human frataxin mutation found in hypertrophic cardiomyopathy. *Mol Genet Metab,* 85, 280-5.

VAUGHN, C. B., WEINSTEIN, R., BOND, B., RICE, R., VAUGHN, R. W., MCKENDRICK, A., AYAD, G., ROCKWELL, M. A. & ROCCHIO,

R. (1987) Ferritin content in human cancerous and noncancerous colonic tissue. *Cancer Invest,* 5, 7-10.

VELASCO-SANCHEZ, D., ARACIL, A., MONTERO, R., MAS, A., JIMENEZ, L., O'CALLAGHAN, M., TONDO, M., CAPDEVILA, A., BLANCH, J., ARTUCH, R. & PINEDA, M. (2010) Combined Therapy with Idebenone and Deferiprone in Patients with Friedreich's Ataxia. *Cerebellum.*

VERGA FALZACAPPA, M. V., VUJIC SPASIC, M., KESSLER, R., STOLTE, J., HENTZE, M. W. & MUCKENTHALER, M. U. (2007) STAT3 mediates hepatic hepcidin expression and its inflammatory stimulation. *Blood,* 109, 353-8.

VIDAL, R., MIRAVALLE, L., GAO, X., BARBEITO, A. G., BARAIBAR, M. A., HEKMATYAR, S. K., WIDEL, M., BANSAL, N., DELISLE, M. B. & GHETTI, B. (2008) Expression of a mutant form of the ferritin light chain gene induces neurodegeneration and iron overload in transgenic mice. *J Neurosci,* 28, 60-7.

WALLACE, D. F., JONES, M. D., PEDERSEN, P., RIVAS, L., SLY, L. I. & SUBRAMANIAM, V. N. (2006) Purification and partial characterisation of recombinant human hepcidin. *Biochimie,* 88, 31-7.

WALLANDER, M. L., LEIBOLD, E. A. & EISENSTEIN, R. S. (2006) Molecular control of vertebrate iron homeostasis by iron regulatory proteins. *Biochim Biophys Acta,* 1763, 668-89.

WANG, T. & CRAIG, E. A. (2008) Binding of yeast frataxin to the scaffold for Fe-S cluster biogenesis, Isu. *J Biol Chem,* 283, 12674-9.

WARD, D. G., ROBERTS, K., STONELAKE, P., GOON, P., ZAMPRONIO, C. G., MARTIN, A., JOHNSON, P. J., IQBAL, T. & TSELEPIS, C. (2008) SELDI-TOF-MS determination of hepcidin in clinical samples using stable isotope labelled hepcidin as an internal standard. *Proteome Sci,* 6, 28.

WARD, P. P., MENDOZA-MENESES, M., CUNNINGHAM, G. A. & CONNEELY, O. M. (2003) Iron status in mice carrying a targeted disruption of lactoferrin. *Mol Cell Biol,* 23, 178-85.

WEST, A. P., JR., BENNETT, M. J., SELLERS, V. M., ANDREWS, N. C., ENNS, C. A. & BJORKMAN, P. J. (2000) Comparison of the interactions of transferrin receptor and transferrin receptor 2 with transferrin and the hereditary hemochromatosis protein HFE. *J Biol Chem,* 275, 38135-8.

WHITE, R. A., BOYDSTON, L. A., BROOKSHIER, T. R., MCNULTY, S. G., NSUMU, N. N., BREWER, B. P. & BLACKMORE, K. (2005) Iron metabolism mutant hbd mice have a deletion in Sec15l1, which has homology to a yeast gene for vesicle docking. *Genomics,* 86, 668-73.

WHITNALL, M., HOWARD, J., PONKA, P. & RICHARDSON, D. R. (2006) A class of iron chelators with a wide spectrum of potent antitumor activity that overcomes resistance to chemotherapeutics. *Proc Natl Acad Sci U S A,* 103, 14901-6.

WHITNALL, M., RAHMANTO, Y. S., SUTAK, R., XU, X., BECKER, E. M., MIKHAEL, M. R., PONKA, P. & RICHARDSON, D. R. (2008) The MCK mouse heart model of Friedreich's ataxia: Alterations in iron-regulated proteins and cardiac hypertrophy are limited by iron chelation. *Proc Natl Acad Sci U S A,* 105, 9757-62.

WHITNALL, M. & RICHARDSON, D. R. (2006) Iron: a new target for pharmacological intervention in neurodegenerative diseases. *Semin Pediatr Neurol,* 13, 186-97.

WHO (2008) Are the number of cancer cases increasing or decreasing in the world? Accessed: 3rd December 2010. http://www.who.int/features/qa/15/en/index.html.

WIEGAND, H., WIRZ, B., SCHWEITZER, A., CAMENISCH, G. P., RODRIGUEZ PEREZ, M. I., GROSS, G., WOESSNER, R., VOGES, R., ARVIDSSON, P. I., FRACKENPOHL, J. & SEEBACH, D. (2002) The outstanding metabolic stability of a 14C-labeled beta-nonapeptide in rats-- in vitro and in vivo pharmacokinetic studies. *Biopharm Drug Dispos,* 23, 251-62.

WILSON, R. B., LYNCH, D. R. & FISCHBECK, K. H. (1998) Normal serum iron and ferritin concentrations in patients with Friedreich's ataxia. *Ann Neurol,* 44, 132-4.

WILSON, R. B. & ROOF, D. M. (1997) Respiratory deficiency due to loss of mitochondrial DNA in yeast lacking the frataxin homologue. *Nat Genet,* 16, 352-7.

WINGERT, R. A., GALLOWAY, J. L., BARUT, B., FOOTT, H., FRAENKEL, P., AXE, J. L., WEBER, G. J., DOOLEY, K., DAVIDSON, A. J., SCHMID, B., PAW, B. H., SHAW, G. C., KINGSLEY, P., PALIS, J., SCHUBERT, H., CHEN, O., KAPLAN, J. & ZON, L. I. (2005) Deficiency of glutaredoxin 5 reveals Fe-S clusters are required for vertebrate haem synthesis. *Nature,* 436, 1035-39.

WOESSMANN, W., CHEN, X. & BORKHARDT, A. (2002) Ras-mediated activation of ERK by cisplatin induces cell death independently of p53 in osteosarcoma and neuroblastoma cell lines. *Cancer Chemother Pharmacol,* 50, 397-404.

WONG, A., YANG, J., CAVADINI, P., GELLERA, C., LONNERDAL, B., TARONI, F. & CORTOPASSI, G. (1999) The Friedreich's ataxia mutation confers cellular sensitivity to oxidant stress which is rescued by chelators of iron and calcium and inhibitors of apoptosis. *Hum Mol Genet,* 8, 425-30.

WONG, C. S., KWOK, J. C. & RICHARDSON, D. R. (2004) PCTH: a novel orally active chelator of the aroylhydrazone class that induces iron excretion from mice. *Biochim Biophys Acta,* 1739, 70-80.

WRIGHTING, D. M. & ANDREWS, N. C. (2006) Interleukin-6 induces hepcidin expression through STAT3. *Blood,* 108, 3204-9.

XU, X., PERSSON, H. L. & RICHARDSON, D. R. (2005) Molecular pharmacology of the interaction of anthracyclines with iron. *Mol Pharmacol,* 68, 261-71.

YANG, C. H., HUANG, C. J., YANG, C. S., CHU, Y. C., CHENG, A. L., WHANG-PENG, J. & YANG, P. C. (2005) Gefitinib reverses chemotherapy resistance in gefitinib-insensitive multidrug resistant cancer cells expressing ATP-binding cassette family protein. *Cancer Res,* 65, 6943-9.

YANG, C. T., YOU, L., UEMATSU, K., YEH, C. C., MCCORMICK, F. & JABLONS, D. M. (2001) p14(ARF) modulates the cytolytic effect of ONYX-015 in mesothelioma cells with wild-type p53. *Cancer Res,* 61, 5959-63.

YOON, T. & COWAN, J. A. (2003) Iron-sulfur cluster biosynthesis. Characterization of frataxin as an iron donor for assembly of [2Fe-2S] clusters in ISU-type proteins. *J Am Chem Soc*, 125, 6078-84.

YOON, T. & COWAN, J. A. (2004) Frataxin-mediated iron delivery to ferrochelatase in the final step of heme biosynthesis. *J Biol Chem*, 279, 25943-6.

YOSHIDA, B. A., SOKOLOFF, M. M., WELCH, D. R. & RINKER-SCHAEFFER, C. W. (2000) Metastasis-suppressor genes: a review and perspective on an emerging field. *J Natl Cancer Inst*, 92, 1717-30.

YU, Y., KALINOWSKI, D. S., KOVACEVIC, Z., SIAFAKAS, A. R., JANSSON, P. J., STEFANI, C., LOVEJOY, D. B., SHARPE, P. C., BERNHARDT, P. V. & RICHARDSON, D. R. (2009) Thiosemicarbazones from the old to new: iron chelators that are more than just ribonucleotide reductase inhibitors. *J Med Chem*, 52, 5271-94.

YU, Y., KOVACEVIC, Z. & RICHARDSON, D. R. (2007) Tuning cell cycle regulation with an iron key. *Cell Cycle*, 6, 1982-94.

YUAN, J., LOVEJOY, D. B. & RICHARDSON, D. R. (2004) Novel di-2-pyridyl-derived iron chelators with marked and selective antitumor activity: in vitro and in vivo assessment. *Blood*, 104, 1450-8.

ZECCA, L., CASELLA, L., ALBERTINI, A., BELLEI, C., ZUCCA, F. A., ENGELEN, M., ZADLO, A., SZEWCZYK, G., ZAREBA, M. & SARNA, T. (2008) Neuromelanin can protect against iron-mediated oxidative damage in system modeling iron overload of brain aging and Parkinson's disease. *J Neurochem*, 106, 1866-75.

ZECCA, L., YOUDIM, M. B., RIEDERER, P., CONNOR, J. R. & CRICHTON, R. R. (2004) Iron, brain ageing and neurodegenerative disorders. *Nat Rev Neurosci*, 5, 863-73.

ZHANG, A. S., ANDERSON, S. A., MEYERS, K. R., HERNANDEZ, C., EISENSTEIN, R. S. & ENNS, C. A. (2007a) Evidence that inhibition of hemojuvelin shedding in response to iron is mediated through neogenin. *J Biol Chem*, 282, 12547-56.

ZHANG, A. S., GAO, J., KOEBERL, D. D. & ENNS, C. A. (2010) The role of hepatocyte hemojuvelin in the regulation of bone morphogenic protein-6 and hepcidin expression in vivo. *J Biol Chem*, 285, 16416-23.

ZHANG, A. S., SHEFTEL, A. D. & PONKA, P. (2005a) Intracellular kinetics of iron in reticulocytes: evidence for endosome involvement in iron targeting to mitochondria. *Blood*, 105, 368-75.

ZHANG, A. S., SHEFTEL, A. D. & PONKA, P. (2006a) The anemia of "haemoglobin-deficit" (hbd/hbd) mice is caused by a defect in transferrin cycling. *Exp Hematol*, 34, 593-8.

ZHANG, P., TCHOU-WONG, K. M. & COSTA, M. (2007b) Egr-1 mediates hypoxia-inducible transcription of the NDRG1 gene through an overlapping Egr-1/Sp1 binding site in the promoter. *Cancer Res*, 67, 9125-33.

ZHANG, Y., LYVER, E. R., KNIGHT, S. A., LESUISSE, E. & DANCIS, A. (2005b) Frataxin and mitochondrial carrier proteins, Mrs3p and Mrs4p, cooperate in providing iron for heme synthesis. *J Biol Chem*, 280, 19794-807

ZHANG, Y., LYVER, E. R., KNIGHT, S. A., PAIN, D., LESUISSE, E. & DANCIS, A. (2006b) Mrs3p, Mrs4p, and frataxin provide iron for Fe-S cluster synthesis in mitochondria. *J Biol Chem,* 281, 22493-502.

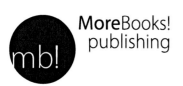
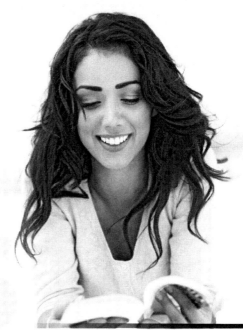

Lightning Source UK Ltd.
Milton Keynes UK
UKOW040243160413

209262UK00001B/105/P

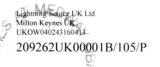